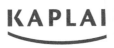

MW00398623

MEDICAL
REFERENCE
GUIDE

···

THE CLINICAL YEARS

Jonathan Phillips, MD
Nancy Herrera-Phillips, MD

This publication is designed to provide accurate and authoritative information in regard to the subject matter covered. It is sold with the understanding that the publisher is not engaged in rendering legal, accounting, or other professional service. If legal advice or other expert assistance is required, the services of a competent professional should be sought.

©2009 Jonathan Phillips, MD and Nancy Herrera-Phillips, MD

Published by Kaplan Publishing, a division of Kaplan, Inc.
1 Liberty Plaza, 24th Floor
New York, NY 10006

Algorithms on pages 4, 7, and 12 are reprinted with permission from the American Heart Association.

Printed in the United States of America

10 9 8 7 6 5 4 3 2 1

ISBN-13: 978-1-4277-9853-4

Contents

Introduction

When entering your clinical years, you are expected to apply your knowledge of the basic sciences. The application of this knowledge in the clinical setting often requires some restructuring of what you already know. *Kaplan's Medical Reference Guide: The Clinical Years* gives you the tools you need to successfully take the step into the clinical setting—whether that is writing a note or treating a patient.

It is important to remember when referring to this book that not all scenarios with similar diagnoses will present the same way. The same goes for treatments. Therefore, the algorithms are provided to guide you through disease management, not patient management. Each patient will respond differently to standard and recommended treatments, thus these treatments may need to be modified accordingly.

You will learn through patient contact that each patient has his or her own unique story, and it is that story that will direct you toward your diagnosis. In order for you to get the complete story, it is important to gain patients' trust and to make them feel comfortable. Remember to have a good bedside manner and be conscious about what you say and the way you present yourself.

As a medical student, you will be asked countless times by your Attending and seniors: "What will/did you find on the physical exam?" "What diagnostic test will you order?" "What is the next step in management?" "What are your differentials?" "What is the treatment?" We've designed this book to take the edge off the anxiety you might feel once you are put on the spot by your Attending or seniors. Realistically speaking, while you are on your clinical rotation, you do not have the time to look up and read pages and pages of information for each of your patients

Medical Reference Guide

before you start rounding on them. We have simplified the information so that you can get the big picture before you start filling in the details.

This book consists of five chapters. The Notes chapter outlines the typical SOAP note and provides examples on how to write one. You will notice throughout your clinical rotations that writing notes is not as simple as it seems. This is an area of the health field that will always have room for improvement. Don't get upset if your Attending doesn't fully approve of your note. Welcome the constructive criticism and learn from it. The Algorithms chapter uses typical scenarios and gives an outline of typical findings, diagnoses, diagnostic tests, management, differential diagnoses, and treatments. The boxes are color-coded to make it easier for you to find exactly what you are looking for without having to read the entire algorithm. The Mnemonics chapter is our collection of mnemonics recommended by medical students over the past few years. These are mnemonics that will be useful while in the hospital. The Abbreviations chapter consists of common abbreviations you may come across while reading through a patient's chart. The abbreviations are also color-coded, so you will know which ones to look at according to your rotation. The Lab Values chapter consists of ranges for some of the common values that you will order. Lastly, the Glossary focuses mostly on terms that may be unfamiliar from the Algorithms chapter.

This reference guide was assembled to help you through the academically and socially challenging clinical years of your medical career. It has the necessary ancillary information that helps with your overall clinical experience. We wish you good luck during your clinical years and encourage you to seize all the learning opportunities they provide!

Dedication

This book is dedicated to our parents Andrea, Luis, Glenn, and Carol, to Rosa (Ta) and our two beautiful girls Amaryllis and Aryana. Thanks for all your support.

Algorithms

Algorithm Categories

Legend

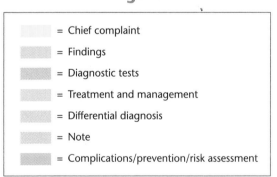

= Chief complaint

= Findings

= Diagnostic tests

= Treatment and management

= Differential diagnosis

= Note

= Complications/prevention/risk assessment

CARDIOLOGY

ACLS Pulseless Arrest

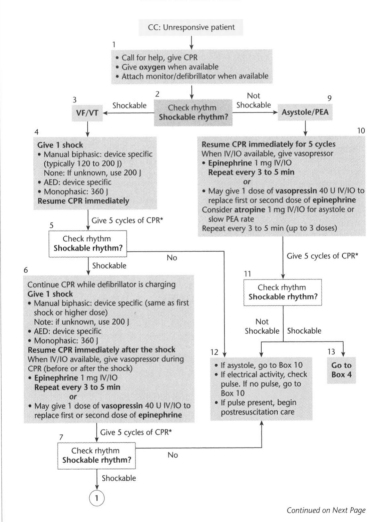

CC: Unresponsive patient

1
- Call for help, give CPR
- Give **oxygen** when available
- Attach monitor/defibrillator when available

2 Check rhythm **Shockable rhythm?**

3 Shockable → **VF/VT**

Not Shockable → **9 Asystole/PEA**

4
Give 1 shock
- Manual biphasic: device specific (typically 120 to 200 J)
  None: If unknown, use 200 J
- AED: device specific
- Monophasic: 360 J
Resume CPR immediately

10
Resume CPR immediately for 5 cycles
When IV/IO available, give vasopressor
- **Epinephrine** 1 mg IV/IO
  Repeat every 3 to 5 min
  or
- May give 1 dose of **vasopressin** 40 U IV/IO to replace first or second dose of **epinephrine**
Consider **atropine** 1 mg IV/IO for asystole or slow PEA rate
Repeat every 3 to 5 min (up to 3 doses)

Give 5 cycles of CPR*

5 Check rhythm **Shockable rhythm?**

No →

Shockable

6
Continue CPR while defibrillator is charging
Give 1 shock
- Manual biphasic: device specific (same as first shock or higher dose)
  Note: if unknown, use 200 J
- AED: device specific
- Monophasic: 360 J
Resume CPR immediately after the shock
When IV/IO available, give vasopressor during CPR (before or after the shock)
- **Epinephrine** 1 mg IV/IO
  Repeat every 3 to 5 min
  or
- May give 1 dose of **vasopressin** 40 U IV/IO to replace first or second dose of **epinephrine**

Give 5 cycles of CPR*

11 Check rhythm **Shockable rhythm?**

Not Shockable | Shockable

12
- If asystole, go to Box 10
- If electrical activity, check pulse. If no pulse, go to Box 10
- If pulse present, begin postresuscitation care

13
Go to Box 4

7 Check rhythm **Shockable rhythm?**

No →

Shockable

(**1**)

Continued on Next Page

CARDIOLOGY

ACLS Pulseless Arrest *(continued)*

8

Continue CPR while defibrillator is charging
Give 1 shock
- Manual biphasic: device specific (same as first shock or higher dose)
  Note: If unknown, use 200 J
- AED: device specific
- Monophasic: 360 J

Resume CPR immediately after the shock
Consider **antiarrhythmics**; give during CPR (before or after the shock)
  amiodarone (300 mg IV/IO once, then consider additional 150 mg IV/IO once) or **lidocaine** (1 to 1.5 mg/kg first dose, then 0.5 to 0.75 mg/kg IV/IO, maximum 3 doses or 3 mg/kg)

Consider **magnesium**, loading dose 1 to 2 g IV/IO for torsades de pointes

After 5 cycles of CPR,* go to Box 5 above

During CPR
- **Push hard and fast (100/min)**
- **Ensure full chest recoil**
- **Minimize interruptions in chest compressions**
- One cycle of CPR: 30 compressions then 2 breaths; 5 cycles ≈ 2 min
- Avoid hyperventilation
- Secure airway and confirm placement

* After an advanced airway is placed, rescuers no longer deliver "cycles" of CPR. Give continous chest compressions without pauses for breaths. Give 8 to 10 breaths/minute. Check rhythm every 2 minutes

- Rotate compressors every 2 minutes with rhythm checks
- Search for and treat possible contributing factors:
  - Hypovolemia
  - Hypoxia
  - Hydrogen ion (acidosis)
  - Hypo-/hyperkalemia
  - Hypoglycemia
  - Hypothermia
  - Toxins
  - Tamponade, cardiac
  - Tension pneumothorax
  - Thrombosis (coronary or pulmonary)
  - Trauma

INTERNAL MEDICINE

Medical Reference Guide

CARDIOLOGY

Atrial Fibrillation

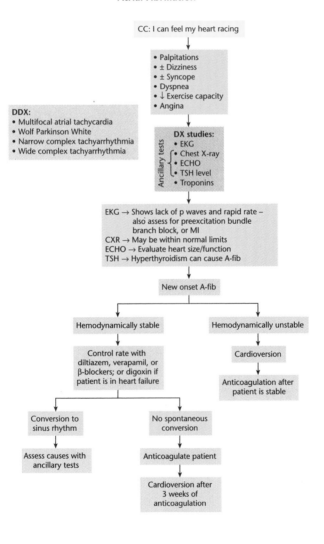

CARDIOLOGY

Bradycardia

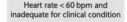

Heart rate < 60 bpm and
inadequate for clinical condition

↓

- Maintain patent **airway;** assist **breathing** as needed
- Give **oxygen**
- Monitor ECG (identify rhythm), blood pressure, oximetry
- Establish IV access

↓

Signs or symptoms of poor perfusion caused by the bradycardia?
(eg, acute altered mental status, ongoing chest pain, hypotension or other signs of shock)

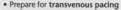

Adequate perfusion | Poor perfusion

Observe/monitor

Reminders
- If pulseless arrest develops, go to
  Pulseless Arrest Algorithm **page 4**
- Search for and treat possible
  contributing factors:
  – Hypovolemia
  – Hypoxia
  – Hydrogen ion (acidosis)
  – Hypo-/hyperkalemia
  – Hypoglycemia
  – Hypothermia
  – Toxins
  – Tamponade, cardiac
  – Tension pneumothorax
  – Thrombosis (coronary or pulmonary)
  – Trauma (hypovolemia, increased ICP)

- **Prepare for transcutaneous pacing;**
  use without delay for high-degree block
  (type II second-degree block or third-
  degree AV block)
- Consider **atropine** 0.5 mg IV while
  awaiting pacer. May repeat to a total
  dose of 3 mg. If ineffective, begin
  pacing
- Consider **epinephrine** (2 to 10 µg/min)
  or **dopamine** (2 to 10 µg/kg per minute)
  infusion while awaiting pacer or if
  pacing ineffective

- Prepare for **transvenous pacing**
- Treat contributing causes
- Consider expert consultation

Reprinted with permission.

2005 American Heart Association Guidelines for Cardiopulmonary Resuscitation
and Emergency Cardiovascular Care, Circulation 2005.

© 2005, American Heart Association

INTERNAL MEDICINE

CARDIOLOGY

Chest Pain Differentials

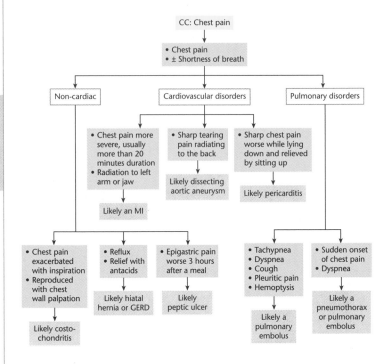

CARDIOLOGY

Congestive Heart Failure

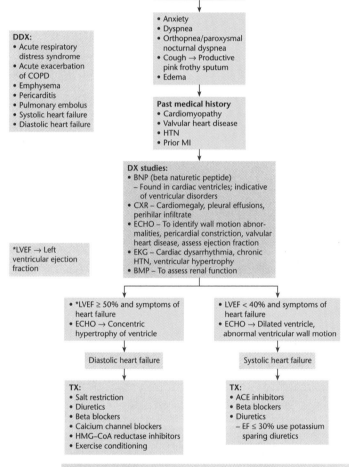

CC: My legs are swelling

- Anxiety
- Dyspnea
- Orthopnea/paroxysmal nocturnal dyspnea
- Cough → Productive pink frothy sputum
- Edema

DDX:
- Acute respiratory distress syndrome
- Acute exacerbation of COPD
- Emphysema
- Pericarditis
- Pulmonary embolus
- Systolic heart failure
- Diastolic heart failure

Past medical history
- Cardiomyopathy
- Valvular heart disease
- HTN
- Prior MI

DX studies:
- BNP (beta naturetic peptide)
  - Found in cardiac ventricles; indicative of ventricular disorders
- CXR – Cardiomegaly, pleural effusions, perihilar infiltrate
- ECHO – To identify wall motion abnormalities, pericardial constriction, valvular heart disease, assess ejection fraction
- EKG – Cardiac dysarrhythmia, chronic HTN, ventricular hypertrophy
- BMP – To assess renal function

*LVEF → Left ventricular ejection fraction

- *LVEF ≥ 50% and symptoms of heart failure
- ECHO → Concentric hypertrophy of ventricle

- LVEF < 40% and symptoms of heart failure
- ECHO → Dilated ventricle, abnormal ventricular wall motion

Diastolic heart failure

Systolic heart failure

TX:
- Salt restriction
- Diuretics
- Beta blockers
- Calcium channel blockers
- HMG–CoA reductase inhibitors
- Exercise conditioning

TX:
- ACE inhibitors
- Beta blockers
- Diuretics
  - EF ≤ 30% use potassium sparing diuretics

NYHA staging system
Class I: Patients have no limitations of activity – no symptoms with ordinary activity
Class II: Mild limitations of activity – no symptoms with mild exertion
Class III: Marked limitation of activities – patients are comfortable at rest
Class IV: Symptoms occur at rest and with any level of physical activity

INTERNAL MEDICINE

CARDIOLOGY

Evaluation of Hypertension

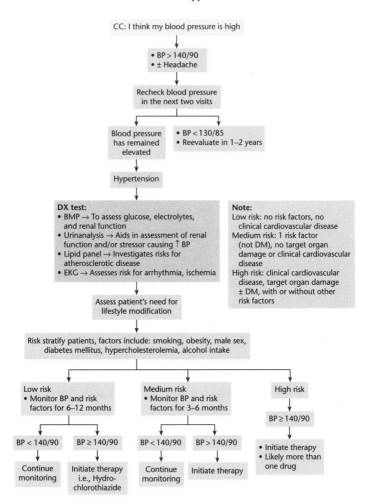

CC: I think my blood pressure is high

↓

- BP > 140/90
- ± Headache

↓

Recheck blood pressure in the next two visits

↓

Blood pressure has remained elevated

- BP < 130/85
- Reevaluate in 1–2 years

↓

Hypertension

↓

DX test:
- BMP → To assess glucose, electrolytes, and renal function
- Urinanalysis → Aids in assessment of renal function and/or stressor causing ↑ BP
- Lipid panel → Investigates risks for atherosclerotic disease
- EKG → Assesses risk for arrhythmia, ischemia

Note:
Low risk: no risk factors, no clinical cardiovascular disease
Medium risk: 1 risk factor (not DM), no target organ damage or clinical cardiovascular disease
High risk: clinical cardiovascular disease, target organ damage ± DM, with or without other risk factors

↓

Assess patient's need for lifestyle modification

↓

Risk stratify patients, factors include: smoking, obesity, male sex, diabetes mellitus, hypercholesterolemia, alcohol intake

↓

Low risk
- Monitor BP and risk factors for 6–12 months

BP < 140/90 → Continue monitoring

BP ≥ 140/90 → Initiate therapy i.e., Hydro-chlorothiazide

Medium risk
- Monitor BP and risk factors for 3–6 months

BP < 140/90 → Continue monitoring

BP > 140/90 → Initiate therapy

High risk

↓

BP ≥ 140/90

↓

- Initiate therapy
- Likely more than one drug

CARDIOLOGY

Myocardial Infarction

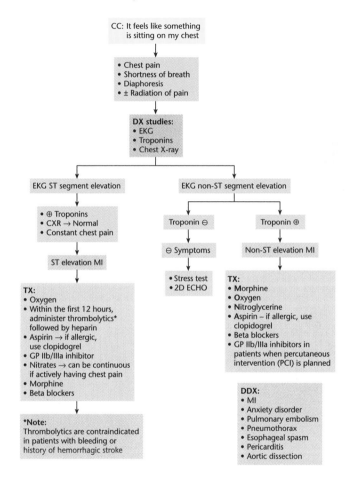

CC: It feels like something is sitting on my chest

- Chest pain
- Shortness of breath
- Diaphoresis
- ± Radiation of pain

DX studies:
- EKG
- Troponins
- Chest X-ray

EKG ST segment elevation

- ⊕ Troponins
- CXR → Normal
- Constant chest pain

ST elevation MI

TX:
- Oxygen
- Within the first 12 hours, administer thrombolytics* followed by heparin
- Aspirin → if allergic, use clopidogrel
- GP IIb/IIIa inhibitor
- Nitrates → can be continuous if actively having chest pain
- Morphine
- Beta blockers

*Note:
Thrombolytics are contraindicated in patients with bleeding or history of hemorrhagic stroke

EKG non-ST segment elevation

Troponin ⊖

⊖ Symptoms

- Stress test
- 2D ECHO

Troponin ⊕

Non-ST elevation MI

TX:
- Morphine
- Oxygen
- Nitroglycerine
- Aspirin – if allergic, use clopidogrel
- Beta blockers
- GP IIb/IIIa inhibitors in patients when percutaneous intervention (PCI) is planned

DDX:
- MI
- Anxiety disorder
- Pulmonary embolism
- Pneumothorax
- Esophageal spasm
- Pericarditis
- Aortic dissection

INTERNAL MEDICINE

CARDIOLOGY

Tachycardia

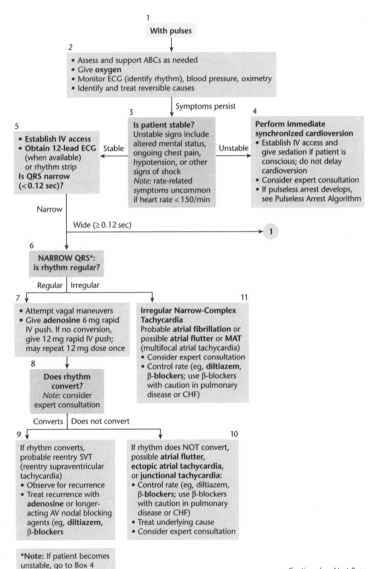

1
With pulses

2
- Assess and support ABCs as needed
- Give **oxygen**
- Monitor ECG (identify rhythm), blood pressure, oximetry
- Identify and treat reversible causes

Symptoms persist

3
Is patient stable?
Unstable signs include altered mental status, ongoing chest pain, hypotension, or other signs of shock
Note: rate-related symptoms uncommon if heart rate < 150/min

4
Perform immediate synchronized cardioversion
- Establish IV access and give sedation if patient is conscious; do not delay cardioversion
- Consider expert consultation
- If pulseless arrest develops, see Pulseless Arrest Algorithm

Unstable

5
- **Establish IV access**
- **Obtain 12-lead ECG** (when available) or rhythm strip
Is QRS narrow (< 0.12 sec)?

Stable

Narrow

Wide (≥ 0.12 sec) → **1**

6
NARROW QRS*: is rhythm regular?

Regular | Irregular

7
- Attempt vagal maneuvers
- Give **adenosine** 6 mg rapid IV push. If no conversion, give 12 mg rapid IV push; may repeat 12 mg dose once

8
Does rhythm convert?
Note: consider expert consultation

Converts | Does not convert

11
Irregular Narrow-Complex Tachycardia
Probable **atrial fibrillation** or possible **atrial flutter** or **MAT** (multifocal atrial tachycardia)
- Consider expert consultation
- Control rate (eg, **diltiazem**, β-**blockers**; use β-blockers with caution in pulmonary disease or CHF)

9
If rhythm converts, probable reentry SVT (reentry supraventricular tachycardia)
- Observe for recurrence
- Treat recurrence with **adenosine** or longer-acting AV nodal blocking agents (eg, **diltiazem**, β-**blockers**

10
If rhythm does NOT convert, possible **atrial flutter**, **ectopic atrial tachycardia**, or **junctional tachycardia**:
- Control rate (eg, diltiazem, β-**blockers**; use β-blockers with caution in pulmonary disease or CHF)
- Treat underlying cause
- Consider expert consultation

*Note: If patient becomes unstable, go to Box 4

Continued on Next Page

Algorithms

CARDIOLOGY

Tachycardia (continued)

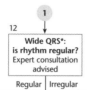

12

Wide QRS*:
is rhythm regular?
Expert consultation
advised

Regular | Irregular

13

If ventricular tachycardia or uncertain rhythm
- **Amiodarone** 150 mg IV over 10 min. Repeat as needed to maximum dose of 2.2 g/24 hours
- Prepare for elective **synchronized cardioversion**

If SVT with aberrancy
- Give **adenosine** (go to Box 7)

14

If atrial fibrillation with aberrancy
- See Irregular Narrow-Complex Tachycardia (Box 11)

If pre-excited atrial fibrillation (AF + WPW)
- Expert consultation advised
- Avoid AV nodal blocking agents (eg, **adenosine, digoxin, diltiazem, verapamil**)
- Consider antiarrhythmics (eg, amiodarone 150 mg IV over 10 min)

If **recurrent polymorphic VT**, see expert consultation

If **torsades de pointes**, give **magnesium** (load with 1–2 g over 5–60 min, then infusion)

During evaluation	Treat contributing factors:	
• Secure, verify airway and vascular access when possible	– Hypovolemia	– Toxins
	– Hypoxia	– Tamponade, cardiac
	– Hydrogen ion (acidosis)	– Tension pneumothorax
• Consider expert consultation	– Hypo-/hyperkalemia	– Thrombosis (coronary or pulmonary)
• Prepare for cardioversion	– Hypoglycemia	– Trauma (hypovolemia)
	– Hypothermia	

Reprinted with permission.

2005 American Heart Association Guidelines for Cardiopulmonary Resuscitation and Emergency Cardiovascular Care, Circulation 2005.

INTERNAL MEDICINE

ENDOCRINOLOGY

Cushings Syndrome

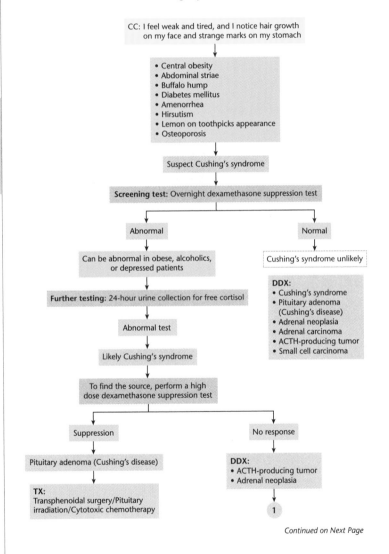

CC: I feel weak and tired, and I notice hair growth on my face and strange marks on my stomach

- Central obesity
- Abdominal striae
- Buffalo hump
- Diabetes mellitus
- Amenorrhea
- Hirsutism
- Lemon on toothpicks appearance
- Osteoporosis

Suspect Cushing's syndrome

Screening test: Overnight dexamethasone suppression test

Abnormal

Normal

Can be abnormal in obese, alcoholics, or depressed patients

Cushing's syndrome unlikely

DDX:
- Cushing's syndrome
- Pituitary adenoma (Cushing's disease)
- Adrenal neoplasia
- Adrenal carcinoma
- ACTH-producing tumor
- Small cell carcinoma

Further testing: 24-hour urine collection for free cortisol

Abnormal test

Likely Cushing's syndrome

To find the source, perform a high dose dexamethasone suppression test

Suppression

No response

Pituitary adenoma (Cushing's disease)

DDX:
- ACTH-producing tumor
- Adrenal neoplasia

TX:
Transphenoidal surgery/Pituitary irradiation/Cytotoxic chemotherapy

1

Continued on Next Page

INTERNAL MEDICINE

ENDOCRINOLOGY

Cushings Syndrome *(continued)*

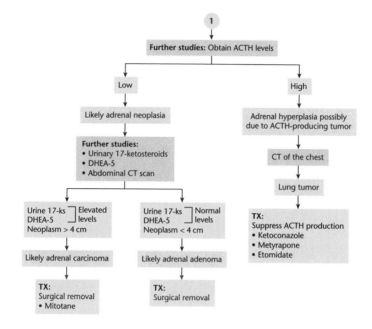

ENDOCRINOLOGY

Diabetes Mellitus

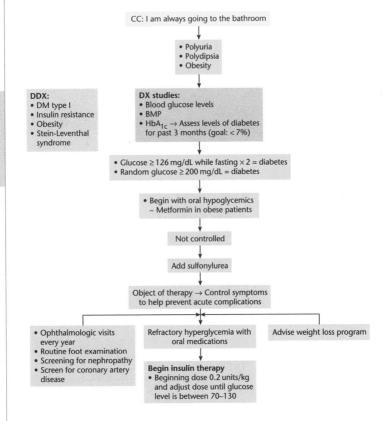

CC: I am always going to the bathroom

- Polyuria
- Polydipsia
- Obesity

DDX:
- DM type I
- Insulin resistance
- Obesity
- Stein-Leventhal syndrome

DX studies:
- Blood glucose levels
- BMP
- HbA_{1c} → Assess levels of diabetes for past 3 months (goal: < 7%)

- Glucose ≥ 126 mg/dL while fasting × 2 = diabetes
- Random glucose ≥ 200 mg/dL = diabetes

- Begin with oral hypoglycemics
  – Metformin in obese patients

Not controlled

Add sulfonylurea

Object of therapy → Control symptoms to help prevent acute complications

- Ophthalmologic visits every year
- Routine foot examination
- Screening for nephropathy
- Screen for coronary artery disease

Refractory hyperglycemia with oral medications

Begin insulin therapy
- Beginning dose 0.2 units/kg and adjust dose until glucose level is between 70–130

Advise weight loss program

Algorithms

ENDOCRINOLOGY

Diabetes Ketoacidosis

CC: Severe abdominal pain and weakness

↓

- Younger patient
- Severe abdominal pain
- Dehydration
- Polyuria
- Polydipsia

↓

Suspect DKA*

↓

*Note:
Think about causes:
- Drugs
- Infections
- Metabolic causes

DX studies:
- BMP (includes glucose)
- ABG
- U/A
- Acetone levels
- Blood culture
- Urine culture
- Urine toxicology

↓

**Note:
If K^+ is normal or low from the beginning, then add K^+ at the beginning of treatment

BMP**:
- ↓ Na^+, ↑ K^+, ↓ Cl^-, ↓ bicarb, ↑ BUN, ↑ Cr, ↑ glucose
- ABG → ↓ pH, ↓ bicarb, ↑ acetone (normal would be negative), ↑ anion gap

↓

TX:
- Initial: Rapid infusion of NS-1-2L
- Initial hourly infusion of insulin @ 0.1 mg/kg/hr (insulin drip)
- Initial bolus of 20 units of insulin
- Empiric antibiotics
- NPO

↓

- Finger stick hourly
- Electrolytes, i.e., BMP, Mg, Phos, K^+ every 2 hours
- Venous blood gas every 2 hours
- Normal saline for 2–4 hours then begin ½ NS
  You can add KCl once K^+ normalizes

↓

- Maintain insulin drip until the bicarb level is normalized and there is no longer ketosis or acetone level is 0
- Discontinue ½ NS and replace with D5½ NS + KCl

↓

- Glucose should now be approximately 200
- Bicarb is normalized

↓

- Start patient on regular insulin
- Discontinue IV infusion after 1–2 hours

↓

Continued on Next Page

INTERNAL MEDICINE

ENDOCRINOLOGY

Diabetes Ketoacidosis *(continued)*

- Start patient on regular insulin
- Discontinue IV infusion after 1–2 hours

- Feed patient
- ↓ or shut off fluids

- Switch the patient to oral antibiotics
- Give patient counseling and educate the patient about DM I
- Place patient on maintenance dose of insulin for home
- Nutritional counseling

Note:

Somogyi effect → Rebound hyperglycemia following an episode of hypoglycemia during sleep. The patient may go to sleep with normal glucose levels, which may drop during the night triggering the release of counter regulatory hormones increasing the amount of glucose in the blood

Dawn phenomenon → High blood glucose levels in the morning requiring an increase in insulin in order to maintain euglycemia

Honeymoon period → A short period of time after the diagnosis of diabetes in which there is a restoration of insulin being produced by the pancreas

ENDOCRINOLOGY

Hypercalcemia

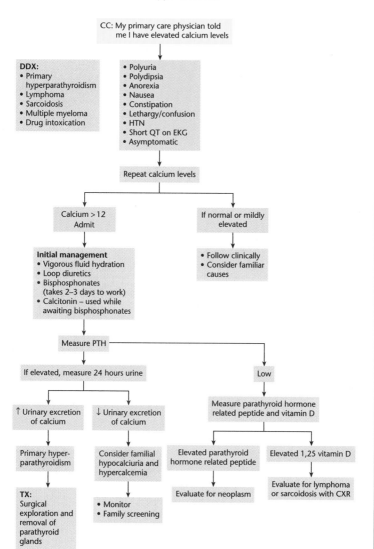

CC: My primary care physician told me I have elevated calcium levels

DDX:
- Primary hyperparathyroidism
- Lymphoma
- Sarcoidosis
- Multiple myeloma
- Drug intoxication

- Polyuria
- Polydipsia
- Anorexia
- Nausea
- Constipation
- Lethargy/confusion
- HTN
- Short QT on EKG
- Asymptomatic

Repeat calcium levels

Calcium >12
Admit

If normal or mildly elevated

Initial management
- Vigorous fluid hydration
- Loop diuretics
- Bisphosphonates (takes 2–3 days to work)
- Calcitonin – used while awaiting bisphosphonates

- Follow clinically
- Consider familiar causes

Measure PTH

If elevated, measure 24 hours urine

Low

↑ Urinary excretion of calcium

↓ Urinary excretion of calcium

Measure parathyroid hormone related peptide and vitamin D

Primary hyper-parathyroidism

Consider familial hypocalciuria and hypercalcemia

Elevated parathyroid hormone related peptide

Elevated 1,25 vitamin D

TX:
Surgical exploration and removal of parathyroid glands

- Monitor
- Family screening

Evaluate for neoplasm

Evaluate for lymphoma or sarcoidosis with CXR

ENDOCRINOLOGY

Hyperthyroidism

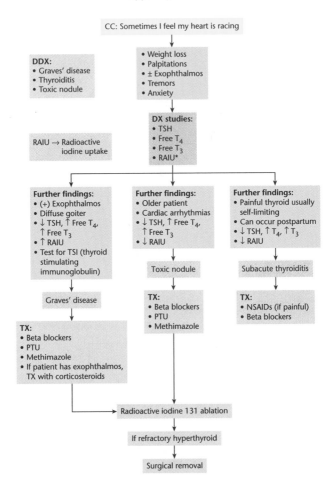

CC: Sometimes I feel my heart is racing

DDX:
- Graves' disease
- Thyroiditis
- Toxic nodule

- Weight loss
- Palpitations
- ± Exophthalmos
- Tremors
- Anxiety

DX studies:
- TSH
- Free T_4
- Free T_3
- RAIU*

RAIU → Radioactive iodine uptake

Further findings:
- (+) Exophthalmos
- Diffuse goiter
- ↓ TSH, ↑ Free T_4, ↑ Free T_3
- ↑ RAIU
- Test for TSI (thyroid stimulating immunoglobulin)

Graves' disease

TX:
- Beta blockers
- PTU
- Methimazole
- If patient has exophthalmos, TX with corticosteroids

Further findings:
- Older patient
- Cardiac arrhythmias
- ↓ TSH, ↑ Free T_4, ↑ Free T_3
- ↓ RAIU

Toxic nodule

TX:
- Beta blockers
- PTU
- Methimazole

Further findings:
- Painful thyroid usually self-limiting
- Can occur postpartum
- ↓ TSH, ↑ T_4, ↑ T_3
- ↓ RAIU

Subacute thyroiditis

TX:
- NSAIDs (if painful)
- Beta blockers

Radioactive iodine 131 ablation

If refractory hyperthyroid

Surgical removal

ENDOCRINOLOGY

Hypothyroidism

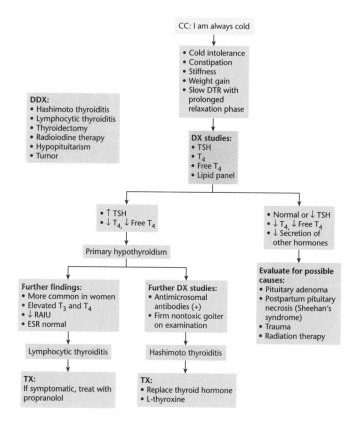

CC: I am always cold

- Cold intolerance
- Constipation
- Stiffness
- Weight gain
- Slow DTR with prolonged relaxation phase

DDX:
- Hashimoto thyroiditis
- Lymphocytic thyroiditis
- Thyroidectomy
- Radioiodine therapy
- Hypopituitarism
- Tumor

DX studies:
- TSH
- T_4
- Free T_4
- Lipid panel

- ↑ TSH
- ↓ T_4, ↓ Free T_4

Primary hypothyroidism

- Normal or ↓ TSH
- ↓ T_4, ↓ Free T_4
- ↓ Secretion of other hormones

Evaluate for possible causes:
- Pituitary adenoma
- Postpartum pituitary necrosis (Sheehan's syndrome)
- Trauma
- Radiation therapy

Further findings:
- More common in women
- Elevated T_3 and T_4
- ↓ RAIU
- ESR normal

Further DX studies:
- Antimicrosomal antibodies (+)
- Firm nontoxic goiter on examination

Lymphocytic thyroiditis

Hashimoto thyroiditis

TX:
If symptomatic, treat with propranolol

TX:
- Replace thyroid hormone
- L-thyroxine

Medical Reference Guide

Achalasia/Cancer of the Esophagus/Schatzki Ring

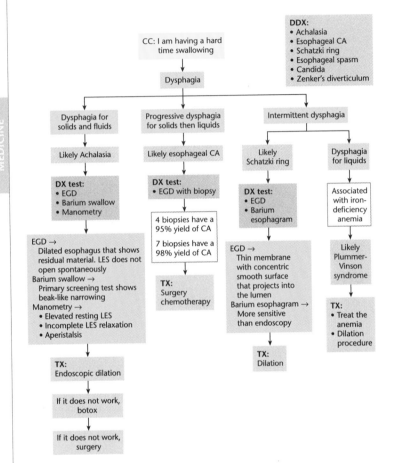

CC: I am having a hard time swallowing

Dysphagia

DDX:
- Achalasia
- Esophageal CA
- Schatzki ring
- Esophageal spasm
- Candida
- Zenker's diverticulum

Dysphagia for solids and fluids

Progressive dysphagia for solids then liquids

Intermittent dysphagia

Likely Achalasia

Likely esophageal CA

Likely Schatzki ring

Dysphagia for liquids

DX test:
- EGD
- Barium swallow
- Manometry

DX test:
- EGD with biopsy

4 biopsies have a 95% yield of CA

7 biopsies have a 98% yield of CA

DX test:
- EGD
- Barium esophagram

Associated with iron-deficiency anemia

EGD →
   Dilated esophagus that shows residual material. LES does not open spontaneously
Barium swallow →
   Primary screening test shows beak-like narrowing
Manometry →
   - Elevated resting LES
   - Incomplete LES relaxation
   - Aperistalsis

TX:
Surgery
chemotherapy

EGD →
   Thin membrane with concentric smooth surface that projects into the lumen
Barium esophagram →
   More sensitive than endoscopy

Likely Plummer-Vinson syndrome

TX:
- Treat the anemia
- Dilation procedure

TX:
Endoscopic dilation

If it does not work, botox

If it does not work, surgery

TX:
Dilation

22

GASTROENTEROLOGY

Colon Carcinoma

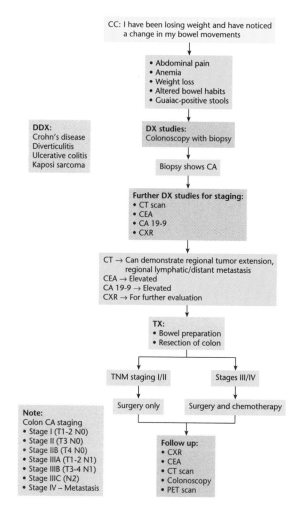

GASTROENTEROLOGY

Constipation

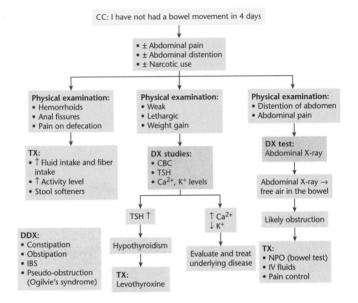

CC: I have not had a bowel movement in 4 days

- ± Abdominal pain
- ± Abdominal distention
- ± Narcotic use

Physical examination:
- Hemorrhoids
- Anal fissures
- Pain on defecation

TX:
- ↑ Fluid intake and fiber intake
- ↑ Activity level
- Stool softeners

DDX:
- Constipation
- Obstipation
- IBS
- Pseudo-obstruction (Ogilvie's syndrome)

Physical examination:
- Weak
- Lethargic
- Weight gain

DX studies:
- CBC
- TSH
- Ca^{2+}, K^+ levels

TSH ↑

Hypothyroidism

TX:
Levothyroxine

↑ Ca^{2+}
↓ K^+

Evaluate and treat underlying disease

Physical examination:
- Distention of abdomen
- Abdominal pain

DX test:
Abdominal X-ray

Abdominal X-ray → free air in the bowel

Likely obstruction

TX:
- NPO (bowel test)
- IV fluids
- Pain control

INTERNAL MEDICINE

GASTROENTEROLOGY

Diffuse Esophageal Spasm/Esophagitis/Zenker's Diverticulum

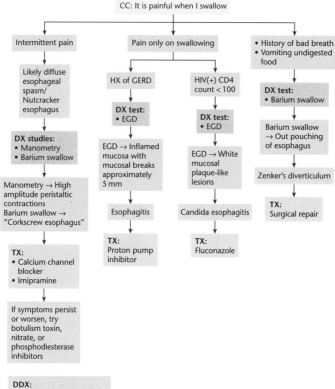

GASTROENTEROLOGY

Divertculitis

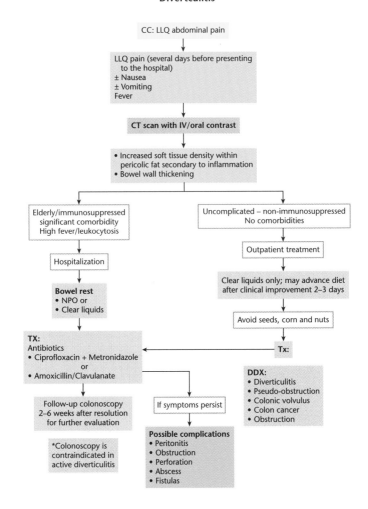

CC: LLQ abdominal pain

LLQ pain (several days before presenting
to the hospital)
± Nausea
± Vomiting
Fever

CT scan with IV/oral contrast

• Increased soft tissue density within
  pericolic fat secondary to inflammation
• Bowel wall thickening

Elderly/immunosuppressed
significant comorbidity
High fever/leukocytosis

Uncomplicated – non-immunosuppressed
No comorbidities

Hospitalization

Outpatient treatment

Clear liquids only; may advance diet
after clinical improvement 2–3 days

Bowel rest
• NPO or
• Clear liquids

Avoid seeds, corn and nuts

TX:
Antibiotics
• Ciprofloxacin + Metronidazole
    or
• Amoxicillin/Clavulanate

Tx:

Follow-up colonoscopy
2–6 weeks after resolution
for further evaluation

If symptoms persist

DDX:
• Diverticulitis
• Pseudo-obstruction
• Colonic volvulus
• Colon cancer
• Obstruction

*Colonoscopy is
contraindicated in
active diverticulitis

Possible complications
• Peritonitis
• Obstruction
• Perforation
• Abscess
• Fistulas

GASTROENTEROLOGY

Inflamatory Bowel Disease

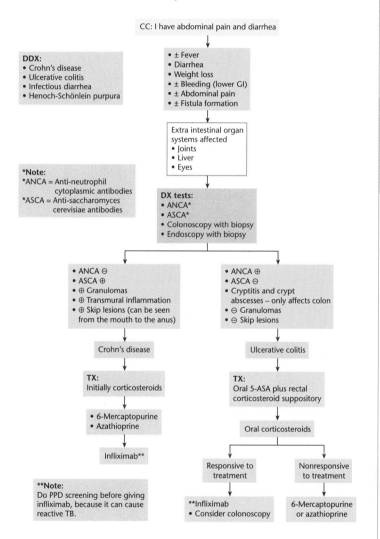

CC: I have abdominal pain and diarrhea

DDX:
- Crohn's disease
- Ulcerative colitis
- Infectious diarrhea
- Henoch-Schönlein purpura

- ± Fever
- Diarrhea
- Weight loss
- ± Bleeding (lower GI)
- ± Abdominal pain
- ± Fistula formation

Extra intestinal organ systems affected
- Joints
- Liver
- Eyes

*Note:
*ANCA = Anti-neutrophil cytoplasmic antibodies
*ASCA = Anti-saccharomyces cerevisiae antibodies

DX tests:
- ANCA*
- ASCA*
- Colonoscopy with biopsy
- Endoscopy with biopsy

- ANCA ⊖
- ASCA ⊕
- ⊕ Granulomas
- ⊕ Transmural inflammation
- ⊕ Skip lesions (can be seen from the mouth to the anus)

- ANCA ⊕
- ASCA ⊖
- Cryptitis and crypt abscesses – only affects colon
- ⊖ Granulomas
- ⊖ Skip lesions

Crohn's disease

Ulcerative colitis

TX:
Initially corticosteroids

TX:
Oral 5-ASA plus rectal corticosteroid suppository

- 6-Mercaptopurine
- Azathioprine

Oral corticosteroids

Infliximab**

Responsive to treatment

Nonresponsive to treatment

**Note:
Do PPD screening before giving infliximab, because it can cause reactive TB.

**Infliximab
- Consider colonoscopy

6-Mercaptopurine or azathioprine

INTERNAL MEDICINE

27

Medical Reference Guide

INTERNAL
MEDICINE

GASTROENTEROLOGY

Malabsorption Syndrome

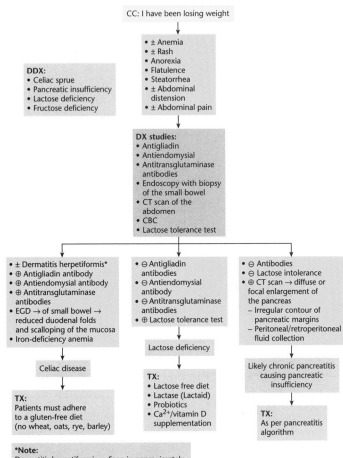

CC: I have been losing weight

DDX:
• Celiac sprue
• Pancreatic insufficiency
• Lactose deficiency
• Fructose deficiency

• ± Anemia
• ± Rash
• Anorexia
• Flatulence
• Steatorrhea
• ± Abdominal distension
• ± Abdominal pain

DX studies:
• Antigliadin
• Antiendomysial
• Antitransglutaminase antibodies
• Endoscopy with biopsy of the small bowel
• CT scan of the abdomen
• CBC
• Lactose tolerance test

• ± Dermatitis herpetiformis*
• ⊕ Antigliadin antibody
• ⊕ Antiendomysial antibody
• ⊕ Antitransglutaminase antibodies
• EGD → of small bowel → reduced duodenal folds and scalloping of the mucosa
• Iron-deficiency anemia

Celiac disease

TX:
Patients must adhere to a gluten-free diet (no wheat, oats, rye, barley)

• ⊖ Antigliadin antibodies
• ⊖ Antiendomysial antibody
• ⊖ Antitransglutaminase antibodies
• ⊕ Lactose tolerance test

Lactose deficiency

TX:
• Lactose free diet
• Lactase (Lactaid)
• Probiotics
• Ca^{2+}/vitamin D supplementation

• ⊖ Antibodies
• ⊖ Lactose intolerance
• ⊕ CT scan → diffuse or focal enlargement of the pancreas
  – Irregular contour of pancreatic margins
  – Peritoneal/retroperitoneal fluid collection

Likely chronic pancreatitis causing pancreatic insufficiency

TX:
As per pancreatitis algorithm

*Note:
Dermatitis herpetiformis → Seen in approximately 10% of the patients; appears as a vesicular rash on the extensor surfaces of the skin

28

GASTROENTEROLOGY

Pancreatitis

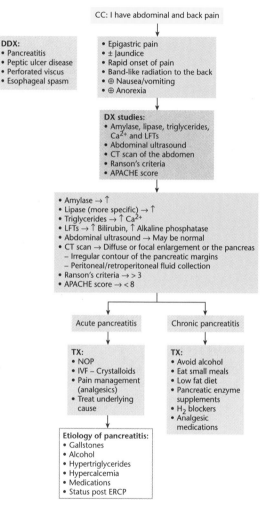

CC: I have abdominal and back pain

DDX:
- Pancreatitis
- Peptic ulcer disease
- Perforated viscus
- Esophageal spasm

- Epigastric pain
- ± Jaundice
- Rapid onset of pain
- Band-like radiation to the back
- ⊕ Nausea/vomiting
- ⊕ Anorexia

DX studies:
- Amylase, lipase, triglycerides, Ca^{2+} and LFTs
- Abdominal ultrasound
- CT scan of the abdomen
- Ranson's criteria
- APACHE score

- Amylase → ↑
- Lipase (more specific) → ↑
- Triglycerides → ↑ Ca^{2+}
- LFTs → ↑ Bilirubin, ↑ Alkaline phosphatase
- Abdominal ultrasound → May be normal
- CT scan → Diffuse or focal enlargement or the pancreas
  - Irregular contour of the pancreatic margins
  - Peritoneal/retroperitoneal fluid collection
- Ranson's criteria → > 3
- APACHE score → < 8

Acute pancreatitis

Chronic pancreatitis

TX:
- NOP
- IVF – Crystalloids
- Pain management (analgesics)
- Treat underlying cause

TX:
- Avoid alcohol
- Eat small meals
- Low fat diet
- Pancreatic enzyme supplements
- H_2 blockers
- Analgesic medications

Etiology of pancreatitis:
- Gallstones
- Alcohol
- Hypertriglycerides
- Hypercalcemia
- Medications
- Status post ERCP

INTERNAL MEDICINE

HEMATOLOGY

Macrocytic Anemia

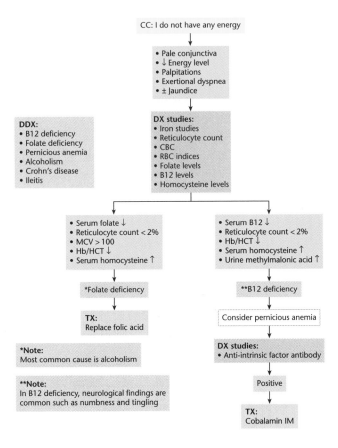

CC: I do not have any energy

- Pale conjunctiva
- ↓ Energy level
- Palpitations
- Exertional dyspnea
- ± Jaundice

DDX:
- B12 deficiency
- Folate deficiency
- Pernicious anemia
- Alcoholism
- Crohn's disease
- Ileitis

DX studies:
- Iron studies
- Reticulocyte count
- CBC
- RBC indices
- Folate levels
- B12 levels
- Homocysteine levels

- Serum folate ↓
- Reticulocyte count < 2%
- MCV > 100
- Hb/HCT ↓
- Serum homocysteine ↑

*Folate deficiency

TX:
Replace folic acid

- Serum B12 ↓
- Reticulocyte count < 2%
- Hb/HCT ↓
- Serum homocysteine ↑
- Urine methylmalonic acid ↑

**B12 deficiency

Consider pernicious anemia

DX studies:
- Anti-intrinsic factor antibody

Positive

TX:
Cobalamin IM

*Note:
Most common cause is alcoholism

**Note:
In B12 deficiency, neurological findings are common such as numbness and tingling

HEMATOLOGY

Microcytic Anemia

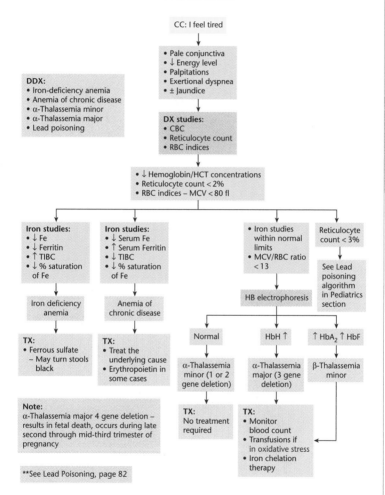

CC: I feel tired

- Pale conjunctiva
- ↓ Energy level
- Palpitations
- Exertional dyspnea
- ± Jaundice

DDX:
- Iron-deficiency anemia
- Anemia of chronic disease
- α-Thalassemia minor
- α-Thalassemia major
- Lead poisoning

DX studies:
- CBC
- Reticulocyte count
- RBC indices

- ↓ Hemoglobin/HCT concentrations
- Reticulocyte count < 2%
- RBC indices – MCV < 80 fl

Iron studies:
- ↓ Fe
- ↓ Ferritin
- ↑ TIBC
- ↓ % saturation of Fe

Iron studies:
- ↓ Serum Fe
- ↑ Serum Ferritin
- ↓ TIBC
- ↓ % saturation of Fe

- Iron studies within normal limits
- MCV/RBC ratio < 13

Reticulocyte count < 3%

See Lead poisoning algorithm in Pediatrics section

HB electrophoresis

Iron deficiency anemia

Anemia of chronic disease

TX:
- Ferrous sulfate – May turn stools black

TX:
- Treat the underlying cause
- Erythropoietin in some cases

Normal

HbH ↑

↑ HbA$_2$ ↑ HbF

α-Thalassemia minor (1 or 2 gene deletion)

α-Thalassemia major (3 gene deletion)

β-Thalassemia minor

Note:
α-Thalassemia major 4 gene deletion – results in fetal death, occurs during late second through mid-third trimester of pregnancy

TX:
No treatment required

TX:
- Monitor blood count
- Transfusions if in oxidative stress
- Iron chelation therapy

**See Lead Poisoning, page 82

HEMATOLOGY

Normocytic Anemia 1

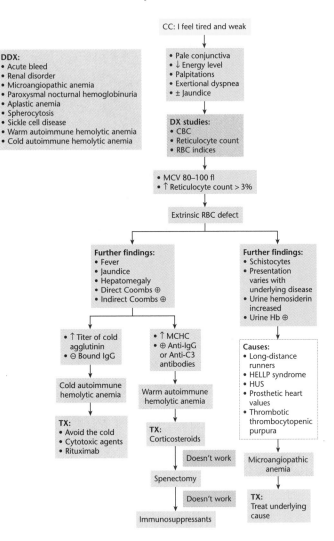

CC: I feel tired and weak

DDX:
- Acute bleed
- Renal disorder
- Microangiopathic anemia
- Paroxysmal nocturnal hemoglobinuria
- Aplastic anemia
- Spherocytosis
- Sickle cell disease
- Warm autoimmune hemolytic anemia
- Cold autoimmune hemolytic anemia

- Pale conjunctiva
- ↓ Energy level
- Palpitations
- Exertional dyspnea
- ± Jaundice

DX studies:
- CBC
- Reticulocyte count
- RBC indices

- MCV 80–100 fl
- ↑ Reticulocyte count > 3%

Extrinsic RBC defect

Further findings:
- Fever
- Jaundice
- Hepatomegaly
- Direct Coombs ⊕
- Indirect Coombs ⊕

Further findings:
- Schistocytes
- Presentation varies with underlying disease
- Urine hemosiderin increased
- Urine Hb ⊕

- ↑ Titer of cold agglutinin
- ⊖ Bound IgG

- ↑ MCHC
- ⊕ Anti-IgG or Anti-C3 antibodies

Causes:
- Long-distance runners
- HELLP syndrome
- HUS
- Prosthetic heart values
- Thrombotic thrombocytopenic purpura

Cold autoimmune hemolytic anemia

Warm autoimmune hemolytic anemia

TX:
- Avoid the cold
- Cytotoxic agents
- Rituximab

TX:
Corticosteroids

Doesn't work

Microangiopathic anemia

Spenectomy

Doesn't work

TX:
Treat underlying cause

Immunosuppressants

INTERNAL MEDICINE

HEMATOLOGY

Normocytic Anemia 2

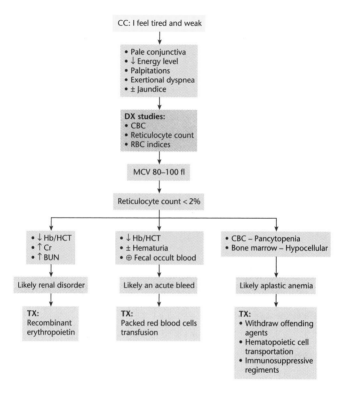

CC: I feel tired and weak

- Pale conjunctiva
- ↓ Energy level
- Palpitations
- Exertional dyspnea
- ± Jaundice

DX studies:
- CBC
- Reticulocyte count
- RBC indices

MCV 80–100 fl

Reticulocyte count < 2%

- ↓ Hb/HCT
- ↑ Cr
- ↑ BUN

Likely renal disorder

TX:
Recombinant erythropoietin

- ↓ Hb/HCT
- ± Hematuria
- ⊕ Fecal occult blood

Likely an acute bleed

TX:
Packed red blood cells transfusion

- CBC – Pancytopenia
- Bone marrow – Hypocellular

Likely aplastic anemia

TX:
- Withdraw offending agents
- Hematopoietic cell transportation
- Immunosuppressive regiments

HEMATOLOGY

Normocytic Anemia 3

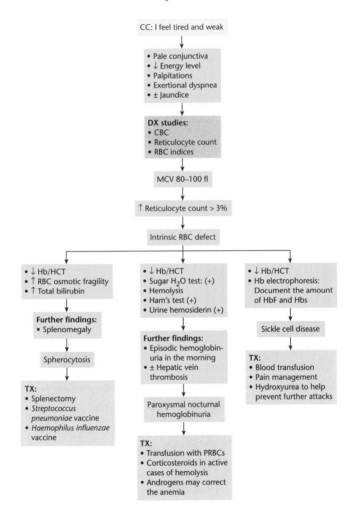

CC: I feel tired and weak

- Pale conjunctiva
- ↓ Energy level
- Palpitations
- Exertional dyspnea
- ± Jaundice

DX studies:
- CBC
- Reticulocyte count
- RBC indices

MCV 80–100 fl

↑ Reticulocyte count > 3%

Intrinsic RBC defect

Branch 1:
- ↓ Hb/HCT
- ↑ RBC osmotic fragility
- ↑ Total bilirubin

Further findings:
- Splenomegaly

Spherocytosis

TX:
- Splenectomy
- *Streptococcus pneumoniae* vaccine
- *Haemophilus influenzae* vaccine

Branch 2:
- ↓ Hb/HCT
- Sugar H_2O test: (+)
- Hemolysis
- Ham's test (+)
- Urine hemosiderin (+)

Further findings:
- Episodic hemoglobin-uria in the morning
- ± Hepatic vein thrombosis

Paroxysmal nocturnal hemoglobinuria

TX:
- Transfusion with PRBCs
- Corticosteroids in active cases of hemolysis
- Androgens may correct the anemia

Branch 3:
- ↓ Hb/HCT
- Hb electrophoresis: Document the amount of HbF and Hbs

Sickle cell disease

TX:
- Blood transfusion
- Pain management
- Hydroxyurea to help prevent further attacks

NEUROLOGY

Coma

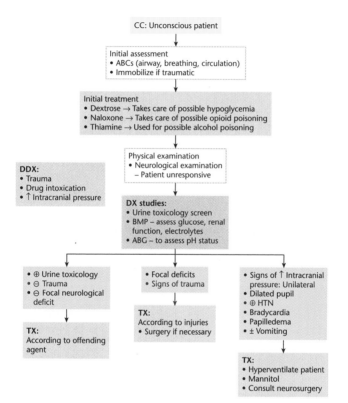

CC: Unconscious patient

Initial assessment
• ABCs (airway, breathing, circulation)
• Immobilize if traumatic

Initial treatment
• Dextrose → Takes care of possible hypoglycemia
• Naloxone → Takes care of possible opioid poisoning
• Thiamine → Used for possible alcohol poisoning

Physical examination
• Neurological examination
  – Patient unresponsive

DDX:
• Trauma
• Drug intoxication
• ↑ Intracranial pressure

DX studies:
• Urine toxicology screen
• BMP – assess glucose, renal function, electrolytes
• ABG – to assess pH status

• ⊕ Urine toxicology
• ⊖ Trauma
• ⊖ Focal neurological deficit

• Focal deficits
• Signs of trauma

• Signs of ↑ Intracranial pressure: Unilateral
• Dilated pupil
• ⊕ HTN
• Bradycardia
• Papilledema
• ± Vomiting

TX:
According to offending agent

TX:
According to injuries
• Surgery if necessary

TX:
• Hyperventilate patient
• Mannitol
• Consult neurosurgery

NEUROLOGY
CVA

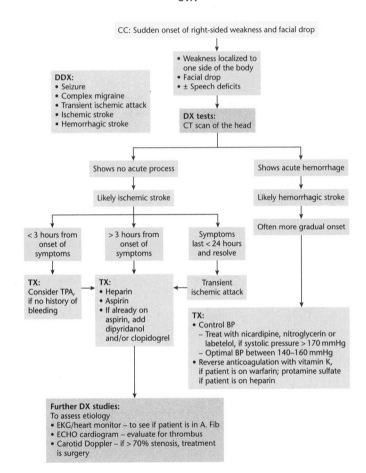

NEUROLOGY

Fatigue

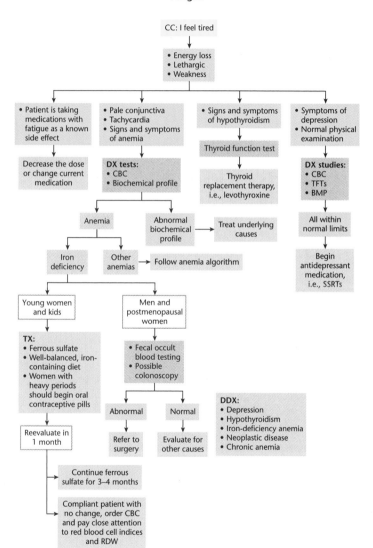

INTERNAL MEDICINE

NEUROLOGY
Head Injury

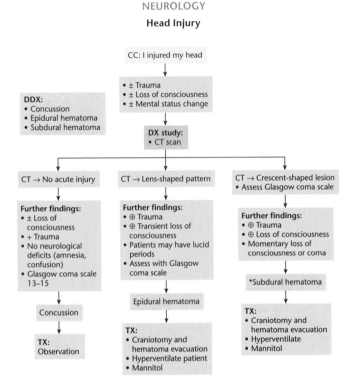

CC: I injured my head

- ± Trauma
- ± Loss of consciousness
- ± Mental status change

DDX:
- Concussion
- Epidural hematoma
- Subdural hematoma

DX study:
- CT scan

CT → No acute injury

Further findings:
- ± Loss of consciousness
- + Trauma
- No neurological deficits (amnesia, confusion)
- Glasgow coma scale 13–15

Concussion

TX: Observation

CT → Lens-shaped pattern

Further findings:
- ⊕ Trauma
- ⊕ Transient loss of consciousness
- Patients may have lucid periods
- Assess with Glasgow coma scale

Epidural hematoma

TX:
- Craniotomy and hematoma evacuation
- Hyperventilate patient
- Mannitol

CT → Crescent-shaped lesion
- Assess Glasgow coma scale

Further findings:
- ⊕ Trauma
- ⊕ Loss of consciousness
- Momentary loss of consciousness or coma

*Subdural hematoma

TX:
- Craniotomy and hematoma evacuation
- Hyperventilate
- Mannitol

Note:
Standard assessment of consciousness used to evaluate patients with suspected concussion:
1. Orientation: Month/Day/Date/Year/Time
2. Immediate memory: 5 words
3. Concentration: String of numbers patient repeats in reverse, such as months in year in reverse order
4. Delayed recall: Using the initial 5 words 5 minutes after immediate memory
5. Neurological screening: Recalls injury, strength, and coordination
6. Exertional maneuvers: 5 sit ups, 5 push ups, 5 knee bends, 40 yard sprint

*Note:
- Acute subdural hematoma 1–2 days after onset of injury
- Subacute subdural hematoma 3–14 days after injury
- Chronic SDH 15 or more days after injury

NEUROLOGY

Headache 1

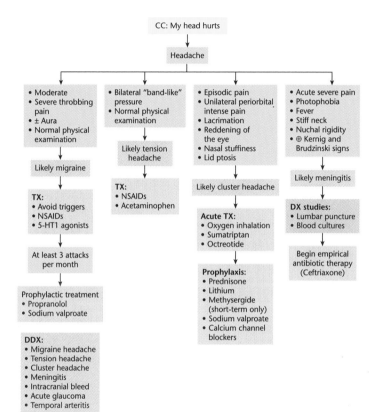

CC: My head hurts

Headache

- Moderate
- Severe throbbing pain
- ± Aura
- Normal physical examination

Likely migraine

TX:
- Avoid triggers
- NSAIDs
- 5-HT1 agonists

At least 3 attacks per month

Prophylactic treatment
- Propranolol
- Sodium valproate

DDX:
- Migraine headache
- Tension headache
- Cluster headache
- Meningitis
- Intracranial bleed
- Acute glaucoma
- Temporal arteritis

- Bilateral "band-like" pressure
- Normal physical examination

Likely tension headache

TX:
- NSAIDs
- Acetaminophen

- Episodic pain
- Unilateral periorbital intense pain
- Lacrimation
- Reddening of the eye
- Nasal stuffiness
- Lid ptosis

Likely cluster headache

Acute TX:
- Oxygen inhalation
- Sumatriptan
- Octreotide

Prophylaxis:
- Prednisone
- Lithium
- Methysergide (short-term only)
- Sodium valproate
- Calcium channel blockers

- Acute severe pain
- Photophobia
- Fever
- Stiff neck
- Nuchal rigidity
- ⊕ Kernig and Brudzinski signs

Likely meningitis

DX studies:
- Lumbar puncture
- Blood cultures

Begin empirical antibiotic therapy (Ceftriaxone)

NEUROLOGY

Headache 2

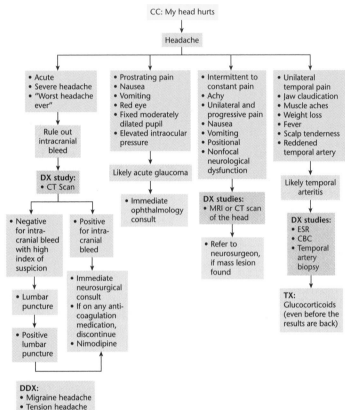

CC: My head hurts

Headache

- Acute
- Severe headache
- "Worst headache ever"

Rule out intracranial bleed

DX study:
- CT Scan

- Negative for intracranial bleed with high index of suspicion

- Positive for intracranial bleed

- Lumbar puncture

- Positive lumbar puncture

- Immediate neurosurgical consult
- If on any anticoagulation medication, discontinue
- Nimodipine

DDX:
- Migraine headache
- Tension headache
- Cluster headache
- Meningitis
- Intracranial bleed
- Acute glaucoma
- Temporal arteritis

- Prostrating pain
- Nausea
- Vomiting
- Red eye
- Fixed moderately dilated pupil
- Elevated intraocular pressure

Likely acute glaucoma

- Immediate ophthalmology consult

- Intermittent to constant pain
- Achy
- Unilateral and progressive pain
- Nausea
- Vomiting
- Positional
- Nonfocal neurological dysfunction

DX studies:
- MRI or CT scan of the head

- Refer to neurosurgeon, if mass lesion found

- Unilateral temporal pain
- Jaw claudication
- Muscle aches
- Weight loss
- Fever
- Scalp tenderness
- Reddened temporal artery

Likely temporal arteritis

DX studies:
- ESR
- CBC
- Temporal artery biopsy

TX:
Glucocorticoids (even before the results are back)

NEUROLOGY

Low Back Pain

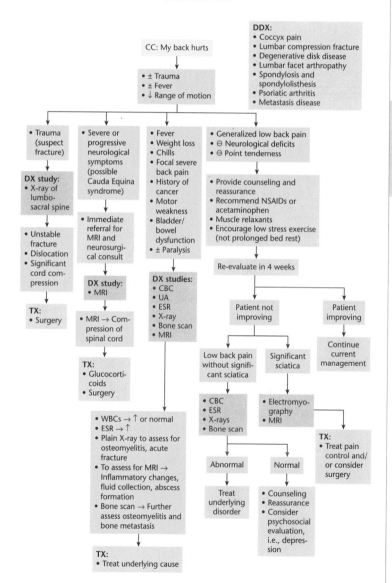

DDX:
- Coccyx pain
- Lumbar compression fracture
- Degenerative disk disease
- Lumbar facet arthropathy
- Spondylosis and spondylolisthesis
- Psoriatic arthritis
- Metastasis disease

CC: My back hurts
- ± Trauma
- ± Fever
- ↓ Range of motion

Trauma (suspect fracture)
- DX study: X-ray of lumbosacral spine
- Unstable fracture
- Dislocation
- Significant cord compression
- TX: Surgery

Severe or progressive neurological symptoms (possible Cauda Equina syndrome)
- Immediate referral for MRI and neurosurgical consult
- DX study: MRI
- MRI → Compression of spinal cord
- TX: Glucocorticoids, Surgery

Fever / Weight loss / Chills / Focal severe back pain / History of cancer / Motor weakness / Bladder/bowel dysfunction / ± Paralysis
- DX studies: CBC, UA, ESR, X-ray, Bone scan, MRI
- WBCs → ↑ or normal
- ESR → ↑
- Plain X-ray to assess for osteomyelitis, acute fracture
- To assess for MRI → Inflammatory changes, fluid collection, abscess formation
- Bone scan → Further assess osteomyelitis and bone metastasis
- TX: Treat underlying cause

Generalized low back pain / ⊖ Neurological deficits / ⊖ Point tenderness
- Provide counseling and reassurance
- Recommend NSAIDs or acetaminophen
- Muscle relaxants
- Encourage low stress exercise (not prolonged bed rest)
- Re-evaluate in 4 weeks

Patient not improving / Patient improving

Patient improving → Continue current management

Patient not improving:
- Low back pain without significant sciatica → CBC, ESR, X-rays, Bone scan → Abnormal / Normal
- Significant sciatica → Electromyography, MRI → TX: Treat pain control and/or consider surgery

Abnormal → Treat underlying disorder

Normal → Counseling, Reassurance, Consider psychosocial evaluation, i.e., depression

INTERNAL
MEDICINE

NEUROLOGY

Vertigo

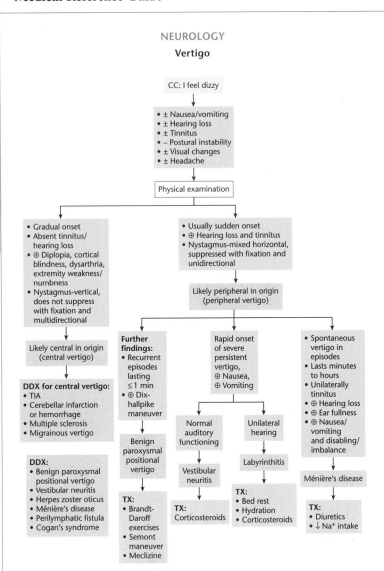

PREVENTATIVE MEDICINE

Preventative Medicine

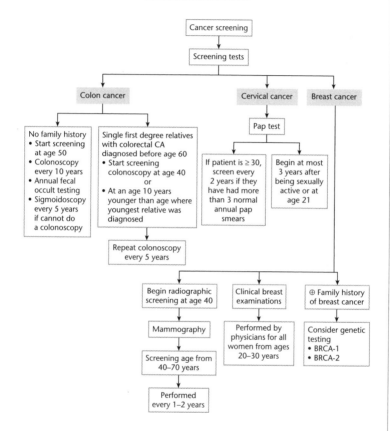

Cancer screening → Screening tests

Colon cancer

No family history
- Start screening at age 50
- Colonoscopy every 10 years
- Annual fecal occult testing
- Sigmoidoscopy every 5 years if cannot do a colonoscopy

Single first degree relatives with colorectal CA diagnosed before age 60
- Start screening colonoscopy at age 40 or
- At an age 10 years younger than age where youngest relative was diagnosed

Repeat colonoscopy every 5 years

Cervical cancer — Pap test

If patient is ≥ 30, screen every 2 years if they have had more than 3 normal annual pap smears

Begin at most 3 years after being sexually active or at age 21

Breast cancer

Begin radiographic screening at age 40 → Mammography → Screening age from 40–70 years → Performed every 1–2 years

Clinical breast examinations → Performed by physicians for all women from ages 20–30 years

⊕ Family history of breast cancer → Consider genetic testing
- BRCA-1
- BRCA-2

INTERNAL MEDICINE

PULMONARY

Bronchiectasis

CC: I have had a cough on and off for years, now it is worse

↓

- Productive cough
- History of repeat lung infections
- Dyspnea
- Wheezing
- Pleuritic chest pain

↓

DDX:
COPD
Chronic bronchitis
Emphysema
Asthma

DX studies:
- CBC → To access for infection
- Immunoglobulins, IgG, IgM, IgA
- CXR
- Sputum cultures → To detect the pathogens
- CT scan (high resolution)
- Pulmonary function test

↓

CBC → ↑ WBC
CXR → Dilated and thickened airways,
   atelectasis (non specific findings)
CT scan (high res) → End on ring shadows
   airway diameter > 1.5 × adjacent vessels
   indicates cylindrical bronchiectasis, cysts
   off the bronchial wall. "Tree in bud pattern."
Pulmonary FX test → Normal to low FVC,
   ↓ FEV, ↓ FEV_1/FVC

↓

Bronchiectasis

TX of acute exacerbation:
- Usually caused by bacterial infection
- Fluoroquinolones
- If hospitalized, IV antibiotics (to cover pseudomonas)
- Corticosteroids
- Extremely severe cases – consider surgery

Preventive TX:
- Patient to maintain adequate oral hydration
- Inhaled corticosteroids
- Prophylactic antibiotics for patients with recurrent exacerbations

PULMONARY

COPD

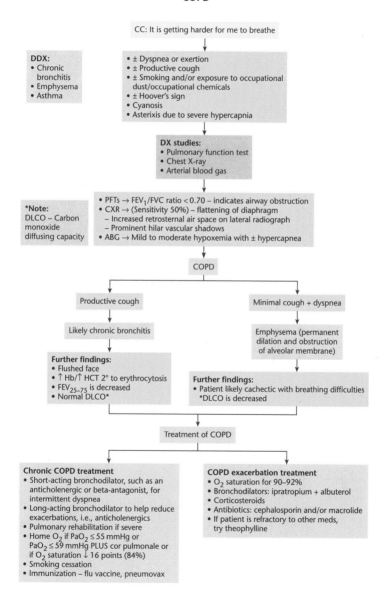

CC: It is getting harder for me to breathe

DDX:
- Chronic bronchitis
- Emphysema
- Asthma

- ± Dyspnea or exertion
- ± Productive cough
- ± Smoking and/or exposure to occupational dust/occupational chemicals
- ± Hoover's sign
- Cyanosis
- Asterixis due to severe hypercapnia

DX studies:
- Pulmonary function test
- Chest X-ray
- Arterial blood gas

*Note:
DLCO – Carbon monoxide diffusing capacity

- PFTs → FEV_1/FVC ratio < 0.70 – indicates airway obstruction
- CXR → (Sensitivity 50%) – flattening of diaphragm
  – Increased retrosternal air space on lateral radiograph
  – Prominent hilar vascular shadows
- ABG → Mild to moderate hypoxemia with ± hypercapnea

COPD

Productive cough

Minimal cough + dyspnea

Likely chronic bronchitis

Emphysema (permanent dilation and obstruction of alveolar membrane)

Further findings:
- Flushed face
- ↑ Hb/↑ HCT 2° to erythrocytosis
- FEV_{25-75} is decreased
- Normal DLCO*

Further findings:
- Patient likely cachectic with breathing difficulties
  *DLCO is decreased

Treatment of COPD

Chronic COPD treatment
- Short-acting bronchodilator, such as an anticholenergic or beta-antagonist, for intermittent dyspnea
- Long-acting bronchodilator to help reduce exacerbations, i.e., anticholenergics
- Pulmonary rehabilitation if severe
- Home O_2 if PaO_2 ≤ 55 mmHg or PaO_2 ≤ 59 mmHg PLUS cor pulmonale or if O_2 saturation ↓ 16 points (84%)
- Smoking cessation
- Immunization – flu vaccine, pneumovax

COPD exacerbation treatment
- O_2 saturation for 90–92%
- Bronchodilators: ipratropium + albuterol
- Corticosteroids
- Antibiotics: cephalosporin and/or macrolide
- If patient is refractory to other meds, try theophylline

PULMONARY

Cough

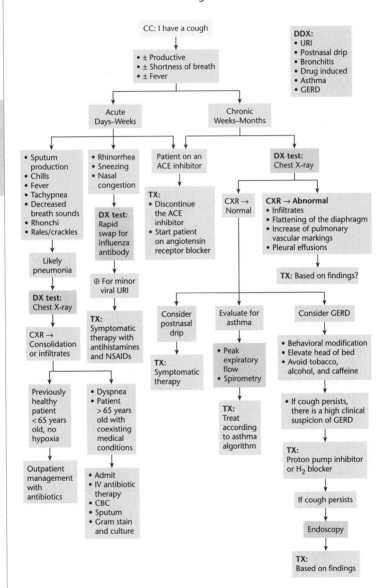

CC: I have a cough

- ± Productive
- ± Shortness of breath
- ± Fever

DDX:
- URI
- Postnasal drip
- Bronchitis
- Drug induced
- Asthma
- GERD

Acute
Days–Weeks

Chronic
Weeks–Months

- Sputum production
- Chills
- Fever
- Tachypnea
- Decreased breath sounds
- Rhonchi
- Rales/crackles

- Rhinorrhea
- Sneezing
- Nasal congestion

Patient on an ACE inhibitor

DX test:
Chest X-ray

Likely pneumonia

DX test:
Rapid swap for influenza antibody

TX:
- Discontinue the ACE inhibitor
- Start patient on angiotensin receptor blocker

CXR →
Normal

CXR → Abnormal
- Infiltrates
- Flattening of the diaphragm
- Increase of pulmonary vascular markings
- Pleural effusions

DX test:
Chest X-ray

⊕ For minor viral URI

TX: Based on findings?

CXR →
Consolidation or infiltrates

TX:
Symptomatic therapy with antihistamines and NSAIDs

Consider postnasal drip

Evaluate for asthma

Consider GERD

Previously healthy patient <65 years old, no hypoxia

- Dyspnea
- Patient >65 years old with coexisting medical conditions

TX:
Symptomatic therapy

- Peak expiratory flow
- Spirometry

- Behavioral modification
- Elevate head of bed
- Avoid tobacco, alcohol, and caffeine

Outpatient management with antibiotics

- Admit
- IV antibiotic therapy
- CBC
- Sputum
- Gram stain and culture

TX:
Treat according to asthma algorithm

- If cough persists, there is a high clinical suspicion of GERD

TX:
Proton pump inhibitor or H_2 blocker

If cough persists

Endoscopy

TX:
Based on findings

INTERNAL MEDICINE

Algorithms

PULMONARY

Pulmonary Thromboembolism

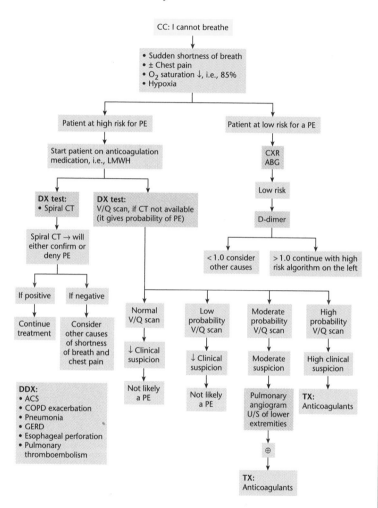

47

RENAL

Urinary Incontinence

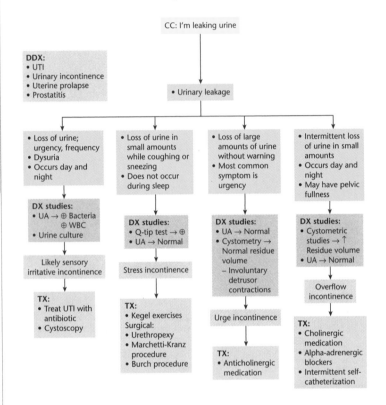

CC: I'm leaking urine

DDX:
- UTI
- Urinary incontinence
- Uterine prolapse
- Prostatitis

- Urinary leakage

- Loss of urine; urgency, frequency
- Dysuria
- Occurs day and night

DX studies:
- UA → ⊕ Bacteria ⊕ WBC
- Urine culture

Likely sensory irritative incontinence

TX:
- Treat UTI with antibiotic
- Cystoscopy

- Loss of urine in small amounts while coughing or sneezing
- Does not occur during sleep

DX studies:
- Q-tip test → ⊕
- UA → Normal

Stress incontinence

TX:
- Kegel exercises
Surgical:
- Urethropexy
- Marchetti-Kranz procedure
- Burch procedure

- Loss of large amounts of urine without warning
- Most common symptom is urgency

DX studies:
- UA → Normal
- Cystometry → Normal residue volume
  - Involuntary detrusor contractions

Urge incontinence

TX:
- Anticholinergic medication

- Intermittent loss of urine in small amounts
- Occurs day and night
- May have pelvic fullness

DX studies:
- Cystometric studies → ↑ Residue volume
- UA → Normal

Overflow incontinence

TX:
- Cholinergic medication
- Alpha-adrenergic blockers
- Intermittent self-catheterization

RENAL

Urinary Tract Infection

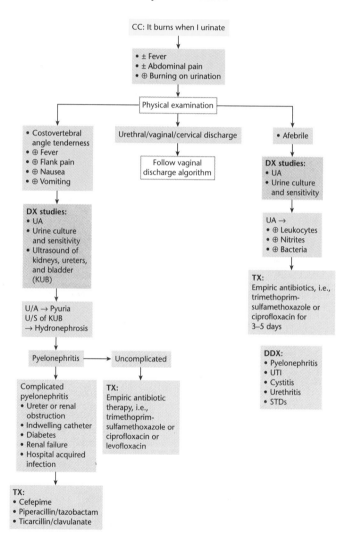

CC: It burns when I urinate

- ± Fever
- ± Abdominal pain
- ⊕ Burning on urination

Physical examination

- Costovertebral angle tenderness
- ⊕ Fever
- ⊕ Flank pain
- ⊕ Nausea
- ⊕ Vomiting

Urethral/vaginal/cervical discharge

Follow vaginal discharge algorithm

- Afebrile

DX studies:
- UA
- Urine culture and sensitivity
- Ultrasound of kidneys, ureters, and bladder (KUB)

U/A → Pyuria
U/S of KUB → Hydronephrosis

Pyelonephritis ⟶ Uncomplicated

Complicated pyelonephritis
- Ureter or renal obstruction
- Indwelling catheter
- Diabetes
- Renal failure
- Hospital acquired infection

TX:
Empiric antibiotic therapy, i.e., trimethoprim-sulfamethoxazole or ciprofloxacin or levofloxacin

TX:
- Cefepime
- Piperacillin/tazobactam
- Ticarcillin/clavulanate

DX studies:
- UA
- Urine culture and sensitivity

UA →
- ⊕ Leukocytes
- ⊕ Nitrites
- ⊕ Bacteria

TX:
Empiric antibiotics, i.e., trimethoprim-sulfamethoxazole or ciprofloxacin for 3–5 days

DDX:
- Pyelonephritis
- UTI
- Cystitis
- Urethritis
- STDs

Medical Reference Guide

RHEUMATOLOGY
Arthiritis

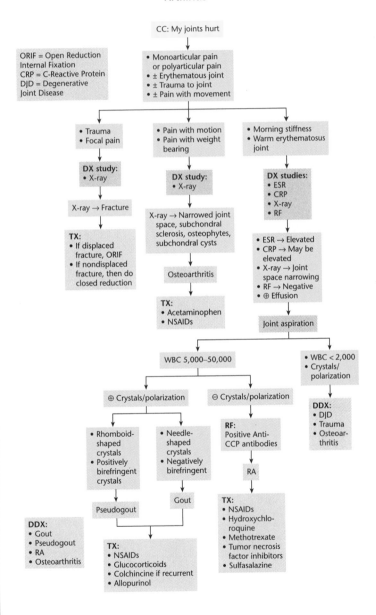

OB/GYN

Abnormal Pap Smear

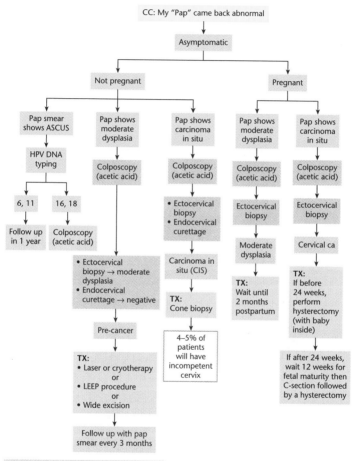

CC: My "Pap" came back abnormal

Asymptomatic

Not pregnant

Pap smear shows ASCUS

HPV DNA typing

6, 11 → Follow up in 1 year

16, 18 → Colposcopy (acetic acid)

Pap shows moderate dysplasia

Colposcopy (acetic acid)

- Ectocervical biopsy → moderate dysplasia
- Endocervical curettage → negative

Pre-cancer

TX:
- Laser or cryotherapy
  or
- LEEP procedure
  or
- Wide excision

Follow up with pap smear every 3 months

Pap shows carcinoma in situ

Colposcopy (acetic acid)

- Ectocervical biopsy
- Endocervical curettage

Carcinoma in situ (CIS)

TX:
Cone biopsy

4–5% of patients will have incompetent cervix

Pregnant

Pap shows moderate dysplasia

Colposcopy (acetic acid)

Ectocervical biopsy

Moderate dysplasia

TX:
Wait until 2 months postpartum

Pap shows carcinoma in situ

Colposcopy (acetic acid)

Ectocervical biopsy

Cervical ca

TX:
If before 24 weeks, perform hysterectomy (with baby inside)

If after 24 weeks, wait 12 weeks for fetal maturity then C-section followed by a hysterectomy

Note:
No endocervical curettage during pregnancy

OB/GYN

OB/GYN

Breast Mass

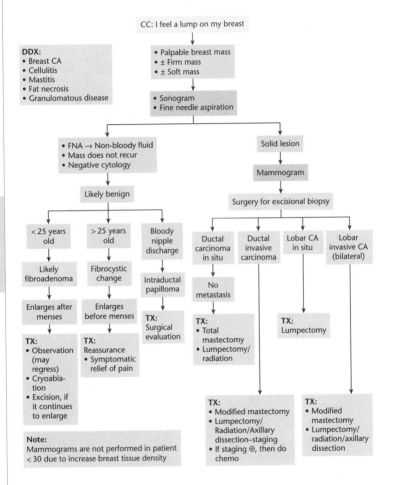

CC: I feel a lump on my breast

DDX:
- Breast CA
- Cellulitis
- Mastitis
- Fat necrosis
- Granulomatous disease

- Palpable breast mass
- ± Firm mass
- ± Soft mass

- Sonogram
- Fine needle aspiration

- FNA → Non-bloody fluid
- Mass does not recur
- Negative cytology

Solid lesion

Mammogram

Likely benign

Surgery for excisional biopsy

< 25 years old

> 25 years old

Bloody nipple discharge

Ductal carcinoma in situ

Ductal invasive carcinoma

Lobar CA in situ

Lobar invasive CA (bilateral)

Likely fibroadenoma

Fibrocystic change

Intraductal papilloma

No metastasis

Enlarges after menses

Enlarges before menses

TX: Surgical evaluation

TX:
- Total mastectomy
- Lumpectomy/ radiation

TX: Lumpectomy

TX:
- Observation (may regress)
- Cryoabla-tion
- Excision, if it continues to enlarge

TX: Reassurance
- Symptomatic relief of pain

TX:
- Modified mastectomy
- Lumpectomy/ Radiation/Axillary dissection–staging
- If staging ⊕, then do chemo

TX:
- Modified mastectomy
- Lumpectomy/ radiation/axillary dissection

Note:
Mammograms are not performed in patient < 30 due to increase breast tissue density

OB/GYN

Algorithms

OB/GYN

Dysmenorrhea

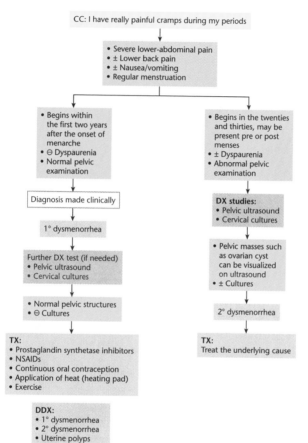

CC: I have really painful cramps during my periods

- Severe lower-abdominal pain
- ± Lower back pain
- ± Nausea/vomiting
- Regular menstruation

- Begins within the first two years after the onset of menarche
- ⊖ Dyspaurenia
- Normal pelvic examination

Diagnosis made clinically

1° dysmenorrhea

Further DX test (if needed)
- Pelvic ultrasound
- Cervical cultures

- Normal pelvic structures
- ⊖ Cultures

TX:
- Prostaglandin synthetase inhibitors
- NSAIDs
- Continuous oral contraception
- Application of heat (heating pad)
- Exercise

DDX:
- 1° dysmenorrhea
- 2° dysmenorrhea
- Uterine polyps
- PID
- Uterine leiomyoma
- Adenomyosis

- Begins in the twenties and thirties, may be present pre or post menses
- ± Dyspaurenia
- Abnormal pelvic examination

DX studies:
- Pelvic ultrasound
- Cervical cultures

- Pelvic masses such as ovarian cyst can be visualized on ultrasound
- ± Cultures

2° dysmenorrhea

TX:
Treat the underlying cause

OB/GYN

Ectopic Pregnancy

CC: I'm having severe abdominal pain, and I'm spotting

DDX:
- Ectopic pregnancy
- PID
- Endometriosis
  (see algorithm, pg 56)
- Ovarian cyst
  (see algorithm, pg 66)
- Appendicitis

- Sudden onset of right-sided abdominal pain
- Vaginal spotting
General examination
  - Flat abdomen
  - Lower-quadrant tenderness
  - Rebound
Speculum examination
  - Closed thick cervix
  - Moderate motion tenderness
  - Slightly enlarged and softened uterus
  - Adnexal tenderness; no palpable mass

- Serum quantitative β-hCG
- Vaginal sonogram
- CBC
- Blood type and Rh

→ Endometriosis

→ Ovarian cyst

- ↑ WBC
- Sonogram may reveal enlarged appendix

⊕ β-hCG

⊖ β-hCG

Vaginal sonogram → No intrauterine gestational sac seen

⊕ Mucopurulent cervical discharge
⊕ Cervical motion tenderness

Appendicitis

TX:
Appendectomy

β-hCG < 1,500 MIU/mL

- β-hCG titer is > 6,000 MIU/mL
- Ectopic mass is > 3.5 cm
- Cardiac activity seen

PT:
Stable

↑ WBC and erythrocyte sedimentation rate

- Follow serial quantitative serum β-hCG (should double every 2 to 3 days)
- Repeat vaginal sonogram

PT:
Hemodynamically unstable

TX:
Laparotomy

- β-hCG titer < 6,000 MIU/mL
- Ectopic mass < 3.5 cm
- No cardiac activity

PID

Possibly an ectopic pregnancy if β-hCG progression is slow or plateaus (may also be a missed abortion)

TX:
Emergency laparotomy

Salpinectomy performed if tube has ruptured or if patient has completed childbearing

TX of choice:
- Methotrexate (compliant patient)
- Administer RhoGAM for Rh-negative patient

TX:
(Antibiotics)
- Cephalosporin and doxycycline
- β-lactamase and doxycycline

Do a follow up quantitative β-hCG

OB/GYN

Endometrial Polyps

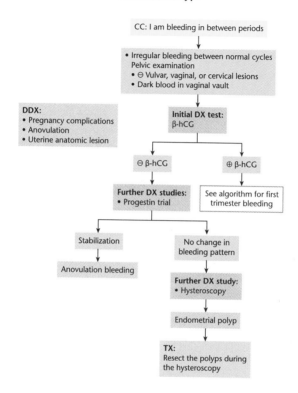

CC: I am bleeding in between periods

- Irregular bleeding between normal cycles
  Pelvic examination
  - ⊖ Vulvar, vaginal, or cervical lesions
  - Dark blood in vaginal vault

DDX:
- Pregnancy complications
- Anovulation
- Uterine anatomic lesion

Initial DX test:
β-hCG

⊖ β-hCG

⊕ β-hCG

Further DX studies:
- Progestin trial

See algorithm for first trimester bleeding

Stabilization

No change in bleeding pattern

Anovulation bleeding

Further DX study:
- Hysteroscopy

Endometrial polyp

TX:
Resect the polyps during the hysteroscopy

Endometriosis

CC: My periods are really heavy

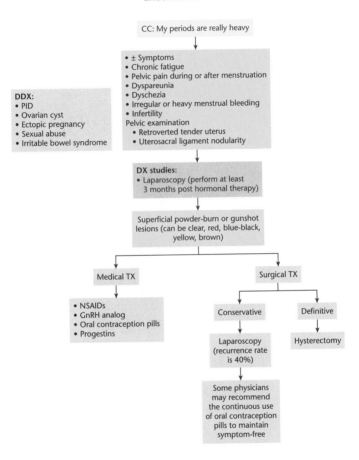

- ± Symptoms
- Chronic fatigue
- Pelvic pain during or after menstruation
- Dyspareunia
- Dyschezia
- Irregular or heavy menstrual bleeding
- Infertility

Pelvic examination
- Retroverted tender uterus
- Uterosacral ligament nodularity

DDX:
- PID
- Ovarian cyst
- Ectopic pregnancy
- Sexual abuse
- Irritable bowel syndrome

DX studies:
- Laparoscopy (perform at least 3 months post hormonal therapy)

Superficial powder-burn or gunshot lesions (can be clear, red, blue-black, yellow, brown)

Medical TX

- NSAIDs
- GnRH analog
- Oral contraception pills
- Progestins

Surgical TX

Conservative

Definitive

Laparoscopy (recurrence rate is 40%)

Hysterectomy

Some physicians may recommend the continuous use of oral contraception pills to maintain symptom-free

OB/GYN

Evaluation of Secondary Amenorrhea

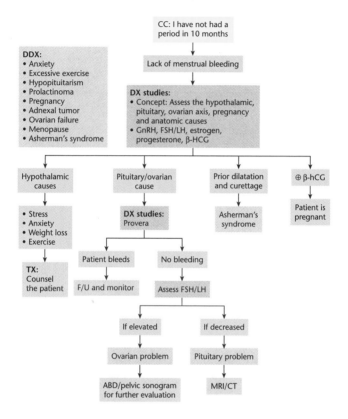

CC: I have not had a period in 10 months

DDX:
- Anxiety
- Excessive exercise
- Hypopituitarism
- Prolactinoma
- Pregnancy
- Adnexal tumor
- Ovarian failure
- Menopause
- Asherman's syndrome

Lack of menstrual bleeding

DX studies:
- Concept: Assess the hypothalamic, pituitary, ovarian axis, pregnancy and anatomic causes
- GnRH, FSH/LH, estrogen, progesterone, β-HCG

Hypothalamic causes
- Stress
- Anxiety
- Weight loss
- Exercise

TX: Counsel the patient

Pituitary/ovarian cause

DX studies: Provera

Patient bleeds → F/U and monitor

No bleeding → Assess FSH/LH

If elevated → Ovarian problem → ABD/pelvic sonogram for further evaluation

If decreased → Pituitary problem → MRI/CT

Prior dilatation and curettage → Asherman's syndrome

⊕ β-hCG → Patient is pregnant

Medical Reference Guide

OB/GYN

Fetal Monitoring

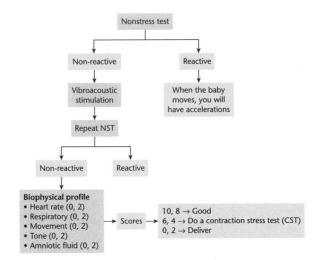

OB/GYN

First Trimester Bleeding Part 1

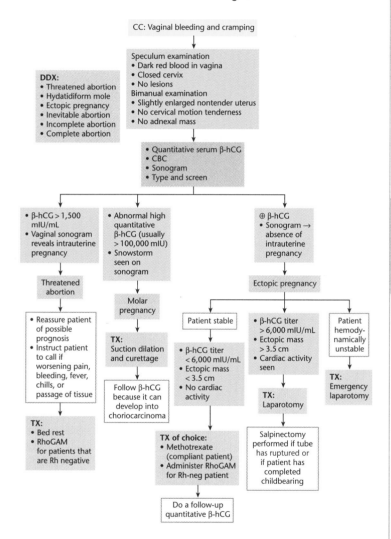

CC: Vaginal bleeding and cramping

Speculum examination
• Dark red blood in vagina
• Closed cervix
• No lesions
Bimanual examination
• Slightly enlarged nontender uterus
• No cervical motion tenderness
• No adnexal mass

DDX:
• Threatened abortion
• Hydatidiform mole
• Ectopic pregnancy
• Inevitable abortion
• Incomplete abortion
• Complete abortion

• Quantitative serum β-hCG
• CBC
• Sonogram
• Type and screen

• β-hCG > 1,500 mIU/mL
• Vaginal sonogram reveals intrauterine pregnancy

• Abnormal high quantitative β-hCG (usually > 100,000 mIU)
• Snowstorm seen on sonogram

⊕ β-hCG
• Sonogram → absence of intrauterine pregnancy

Threatened abortion

Molar pregnancy

Ectopic pregnancy

• Reassure patient of possible prognosis
• Instruct patient to call if worsening pain, bleeding, fever, chills, or passage of tissue

TX:
Suction dilation and curettage

Patient stable

• β-hCG titer > 6,000 mIU/mL
• Ectopic mass > 3.5 cm
• Cardiac activity seen

Patient hemodynamically unstable

Follow β-hCG because it can develop into choriocarcinoma

• β-hCG titer < 6,000 mIU/mL
• Ectopic mass < 3.5 cm
• No cardiac activity

TX:
Laparotomy

TX:
Emergency laparotomy

TX:
• Bed rest
• RhoGAM for patients that are Rh negative

TX of choice:
• Methotrexate (compliant patient)
• Administer RhoGAM for Rh-neg patient

Salpinectomy performed if tube has ruptured or if patient has completed childbearing

Do a follow-up quantitative β-hCG

OB/GYN

First Trimester Bleeding Part 2

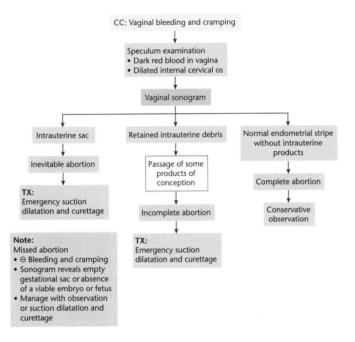

CC: Vaginal bleeding and cramping

Speculum examination
- Dark red blood in vagina
- Dilated internal cervical os

Vaginal sonogram

Intrauterine sac
→ Inevitable abortion

TX:
Emergency suction
dilatation and curettage

Note:
Missed abortion
- ⊖ Bleeding and cramping
- Sonogram reveals empty gestational sac or absence of a viable embryo or fetus
- Manage with observation or suction dilatation and curettage

Retained intrauterine debris
→ Passage of some products of conception
→ Incomplete abortion

TX:
Emergency suction
dilatation and curettage

Normal endometrial stripe without intrauterine products
→ Complete abortion
→ Conservative observation

Gestational Diabetes

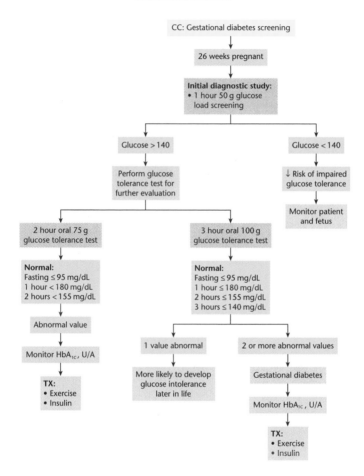

OB/GYN

Gonorrhea and Chlamydia

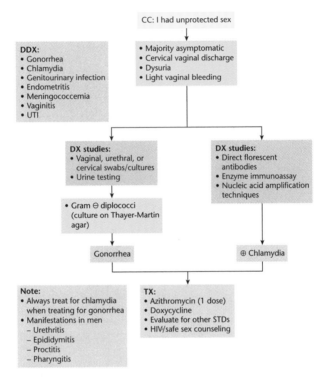

CC: I had unprotected sex

- Majority asymptomatic
- Cervical vaginal discharge
- Dysuria
- Light vaginal bleeding

DDX:
- Gonorrhea
- Chlamydia
- Genitourinary infection
- Endometritis
- Meningococcemia
- Vaginitis
- UTI

DX studies:
- Vaginal, urethral, or cervical swabs/cultures
- Urine testing

- Gram ⊖ diplococci (culture on Thayer-Martin agar)

Gonorrhea

DX studies:
- Direct florescent antibodies
- Enzyme immunoassay
- Nucleic acid amplification techniques

⊕ Chlamydia

Note:
- Always treat for chlamydia when treating for gonorrhea
- Manifestations in men
  - Urethritis
  - Epididymitis
  - Proctitis
  - Pharyngitis

TX:
- Azithromycin (1 dose)
- Doxycycline
- Evaluate for other STDs
- HIV/safe sex counseling

OB/GYN

Hypertension in Pregnancy

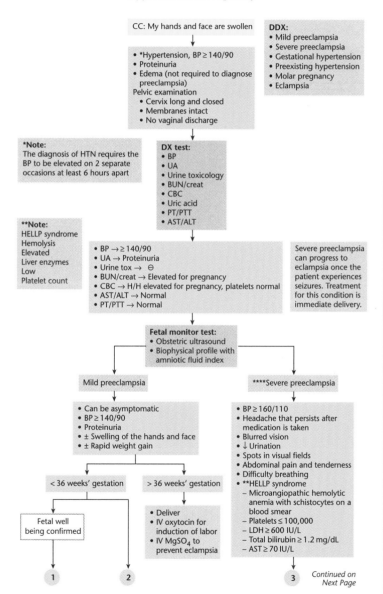

CC: My hands and face are swollen

DDX:
- Mild preeclampsia
- Severe preeclampsia
- Gestational hypertension
- Preexisting hypertension
- Molar pregnancy
- Eclampsia

- *Hypertension, BP ≥ 140/90
- Proteinuria
- Edema (not required to diagnose preeclampsia)
Pelvic examination
  - Cervix long and closed
  - Membranes intact
  - No vaginal discharge

*Note:
The diagnosis of HTN requires the BP to be elevated on 2 separate occasions at least 6 hours apart

DX test:
- BP
- UA
- Urine toxicology
- BUN/creat
- CBC
- Uric acid
- PT/PTT
- AST/ALT

**Note:
HELLP syndrome
Hemolysis
Elevated
Liver enzymes
Low
Platelet count

- BP → ≥ 140/90
- UA → Proteinuria
- Urine tox → ⊖
- BUN/creat → Elevated for pregnancy
- CBC → H/H elevated for pregnancy, platelets normal
- AST/ALT → Normal
- PT/PTT → Normal

Severe preeclampsia can progress to eclampsia once the patient experiences seizures. Treatment for this condition is immediate delivery.

Fetal monitor test:
- Obstetric ultrasound
- Biophysical profile with amniotic fluid index

Mild preeclampsia

****Severe preeclampsia

- Can be asymptomatic
- BP ≥ 140/90
- Proteinuria
- ± Swelling of the hands and face
- ± Rapid weight gain

- BP ≥ 160/110
- Headache that persists after medication is taken
- Blurred vision
- ↓ Urination
- Spots in visual fields
- Abdominal pain and tenderness
- Difficulty breathing
- **HELLP syndrome
  - Microangiopathic hemolytic anemia with schistocytes on a blood smear
  - Platelets ≤ 100,000
  - LDH ≥ 600 IU/L
  - Total bilirubin ≥ 1.2 mg/dL
  - AST ≥ 70 IU/L

< 36 weeks' gestation

> 36 weeks' gestation

Fetal well being confirmed

- Deliver
- IV oxytocin for induction of labor
- IV MgSO$_4$ to prevent eclampsia

1

2

3

Continued on Next Page

Hypertension in Pregnancy *(continued)*

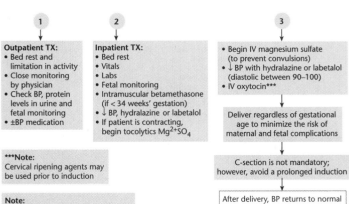

1

Outpatient TX:
- Bed rest and limitation in activity
- Close monitoring by physician
- Check BP, protein levels in urine and fetal monitoring
- ±BP medication

2

Inpatient TX:
- Bed rest
- Vitals
- Labs
- Fetal monitoring
- Intramuscular betamethasone (if < 34 weeks' gestation)
- ↓ BP, hydralazine or labetalol
- If patient is contracting, begin tocolytics $Mg^{2+}SO_4$

3

- Begin IV magnesium sulfate (to prevent convulsions)
- ↓ BP with hydralazine or labetalol (diastolic between 90–100)
- IV oxytocin***

Deliver regardless of gestational age to minimize the risk of maternal and fetal complications

C-section is not mandatory; however, avoid a prolonged induction

After delivery, BP returns to normal after a few days or weeks

***Note:
Cervical ripening agents may be used prior to induction

Note:
All women with preeclampsia should deliver by 40 weeks' gestation

Intrauterine Growth Restriction

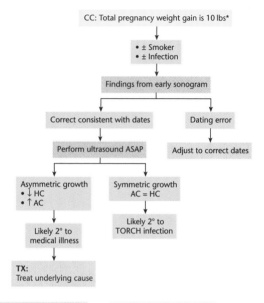

CC: Total pregnancy weight gain is 10 lbs*

↓

- ± Smoker
- ± Infection

↓

Findings from early sonogram

↓

Correct consistent with dates → Perform ultrasound ASAP

Dating error → Adjust to correct dates

Asymmetric growth
- ↓ HC
- ↑ AC

↓

Likely 2° to medical illness

↓

TX:
Treat underlying cause

Symmetric growth
AC = HC

↓

Likely 2° to TORCH infection

HC = Head circumference
AC = Abdominal circumference

Causes:
Maternal:
- Chronic HTN
- Pregnancy-associated HTN
- Smoking
- Substance abuse
- Infection
Placental:
- Placental anomalies
- Twin/twin transfusion
- Multiple gestation

*Note:
Normal pregnancy weight gain is 5 lbs in the first 20 weeks and 1 lb per week in the last 20 weeks

OB/GYN

Medical Reference Guide

OB/GYN

Ovarian Cyst

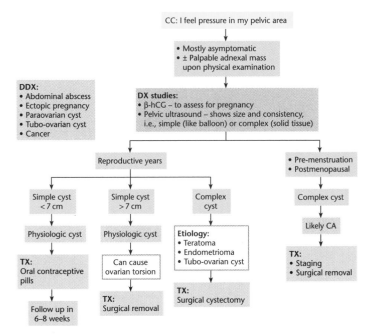

CC: I feel pressure in my pelvic area

- Mostly asymptomatic
- ± Palpable adnexal mass upon physical examination

DDX:
- Abdominal abscess
- Ectopic pregnancy
- Paraovarian cyst
- Tubo-ovarian cyst
- Cancer

DX studies:
- β-hCG – to assess for pregnancy
- Pelvic ultrasound – shows size and consistency, i.e., simple (like balloon) or complex (solid tissue)

Reproductive years

- Pre-menstruation
- Postmenopausal

Simple cyst <7 cm → Physiologic cyst → **TX:** Oral contraceptive pills → Follow up in 6–8 weeks

Simple cyst >7 cm → Physiologic cyst → Can cause ovarian torsion → **TX:** Surgical removal

Complex cyst → **Etiology:** • Teratoma • Endometrioma • Tubo-ovarian cyst → **TX:** Surgical cystectomy

Complex cyst → Likely CA → **TX:** • Staging • Surgical removal

OB/GYN

OB/GYN

Pelvic Inflammatory Disease

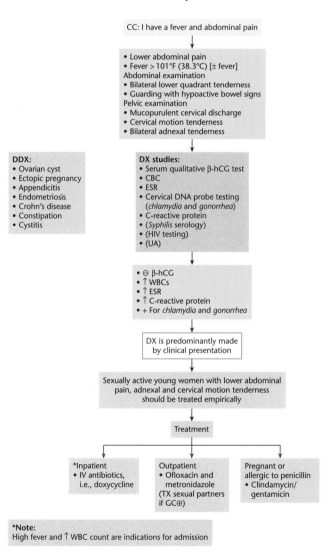

CC: I have a fever and abdominal pain

- Lower abdominal pain
- Fever > 101°F (38.3°C) [± fever]
Abdominal examination
- Bilateral lower quadrant tenderness
- Guarding with hypoactive bowel signs
Pelvic examination
- Mucopurulent cervical discharge
- Cervical motion tenderness
- Bilateral adnexal tenderness

DDX:
- Ovarian cyst
- Ectopic pregnancy
- Appendicitis
- Endometriosis
- Crohn's disease
- Constipation
- Cystitis

DX studies:
- Serum qualitative β-hCG test
- CBC
- ESR
- Cervical DNA probe testing (*chlamydia* and *gonorrhea*)
- C-reactive protein
- (*Syphilis* serology)
- (HIV testing)
- (UA)

- ⊖ β-hCG
- ↑ WBCs
- ↑ ESR
- ↑ C-reactive protein
- + For *chlamydia* and *gonorrhea*

DX is predominantly made by clinical presentation

Sexually active young women with lower abdominal pain, adnexal and cervical motion tenderness should be treated empirically

Treatment

*Inpatient
- IV antibiotics, i.e., doxycycline

Outpatient
- Ofloxacin and metronidazole (TX sexual partners if GC⊕)

Pregnant or allergic to penicillin
- Clindamycin/ gentamicin

*Note:
High fever and ↑ WBC count are indications for admission

OB/GYN

Placenta Previa

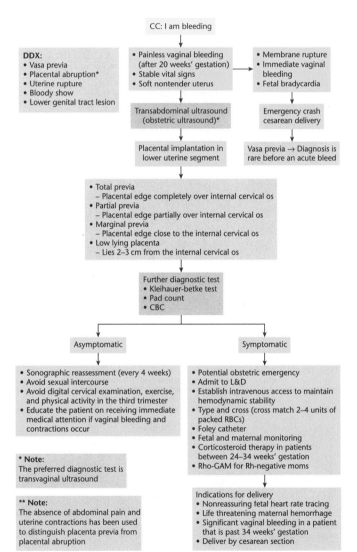

CC: I am bleeding

DDX:
- Vasa previa
- Placental abruption*
- Uterine rupture
- Bloody show
- Lower genital tract lesion

- Painless vaginal bleeding (after 20 weeks' gestation)
- Stable vital signs
- Soft nontender uterus

- Membrane rupture
- Immediate vaginal bleeding
- Fetal bradycardia

Transabdominal ultrasound (obstetric ultrasound)*

Emergency crash cesarean delivery

Placental implantation in lower uterine segment

Vasa previa → Diagnosis is rare before an acute bleed

- Total previa
  - Placental edge completely over internal cervical os
- Partial previa
  - Placental edge partially over internal cervical os
- Marginal previa
  - Placental edge close to the internal cervical os
- Low lying placenta
  - Lies 2–3 cm from the internal cervical os

Further diagnostic test
- Kleihauer-betke test
- Pad count
- CBC

Asymptomatic

Symptomatic

- Sonographic reassessment (every 4 weeks)
- Avoid sexual intercourse
- Avoid digital cervical examination, exercise, and physical activity in the third trimester
- Educate the patient on receiving immediate medical attention if vaginal bleeding and contractions occur

- Potential obstetric emergency
- Admit to L&D
- Establish intravenous access to maintain hemodynamic stability
- Type and cross (cross match 2–4 units of packed RBCs)
- Foley catheter
- Fetal and maternal monitoring
- Corticosteroid therapy in patients between 24–34 weeks' gestation
- Rho-GAM for Rh-negative moms

* Note:
The preferred diagnostic test is transvaginal ultrasound

** Note:
The absence of abdominal pain and uterine contractions has been used to distinguish placenta previa from placental abruption

Indications for delivery
- Nonreassuring fetal heart rate tracing
- Life threatening maternal hemorrhage
- Significant vaginal bleeding in a patient that is past 34 weeks' gestation
- Deliver by cesarean section

OB/GYN

OB/GYN

Placental Abruption

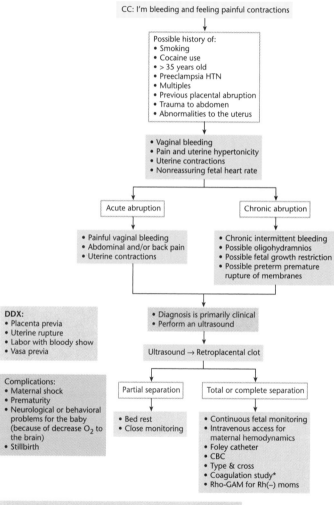

CC: I'm bleeding and feeling painful contractions

Possible history of:
- Smoking
- Cocaine use
- > 35 years old
- Preeclampsia HTN
- Multiples
- Previous placental abruption
- Trauma to abdomen
- Abnormalities to the uterus

- Vaginal bleeding
- Pain and uterine hypertonicity
- Uterine contractions
- Nonreassuring fetal heart rate

Acute abruption
- Painful vaginal bleeding
- Abdominal and/or back pain
- Uterine contractions

Chronic abruption
- Chronic intermittent bleeding
- Possible oligohydramnios
- Possible fetal growth restriction
- Possible preterm premature rupture of membranes

DDX:
- Placenta previa
- Uterine rupture
- Labor with bloody show
- Vasa previa

Complications:
- Maternal shock
- Prematurity
- Neurological or behavioral problems for the baby (because of decrease O_2 to the brain)
- Stillbirth

- Diagnosis is primarily clinical
- Perform an ultrasound

Ultrasound → Retroplacental clot

Partial separation
- Bed rest
- Close monitoring

Total or complete separation
- Continuous fetal monitoring
- Intravenous access for maternal hemodynamics
- Foley catheter
- CBC
- Type & cross
- Coagulation study*
- Rho-GAM for Rh(−) moms

Note:
Fresh frozen plasma, cryoprecipitate and platelets should be available
- Placental abruption is confirmed after delivery

OB/GYN

Postpartum Hemorrhage

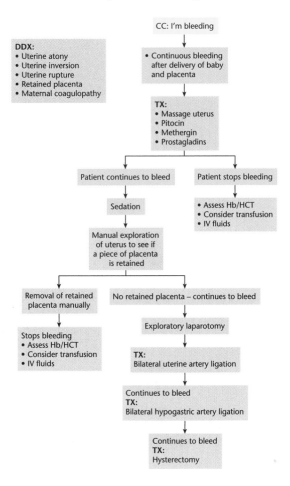

CC: I'm bleeding

DDX:
- Uterine atony
- Uterine inversion
- Uterine rupture
- Retained placenta
- Maternal coagulopathy

• Continuous bleeding after delivery of baby and placenta

TX:
- Massage uterus
- Pitocin
- Methergin
- Prostagladins

Patient continues to bleed

Patient stops bleeding

Sedation

- Assess Hb/HCT
- Consider transfusion
- IV fluids

Manual exploration of uterus to see if a piece of placenta is retained

Removal of retained placenta manually

No retained placenta – continues to bleed

Stops bleeding
- Assess Hb/HCT
- Consider transfusion
- IV fluids

Exploratory laparotomy

TX:
Bilateral uterine artery ligation

Continues to bleed
TX:
Bilateral hypogastric artery ligation

Continues to bleed
TX:
Hysterectomy

OB/GYN

RhoGAM

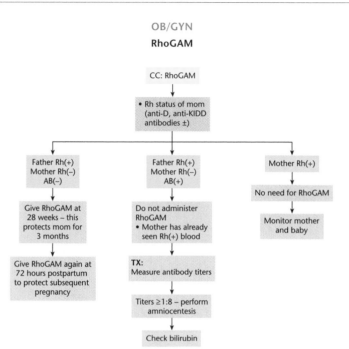

CC: RhoGAM

↓

- Rh status of mom (anti-D, anti-KIDD antibodies ±)

Father Rh(+)
Mother Rh(−)
AB(−)

↓

Give RhoGAM at 28 weeks – this protects mom for 3 months

↓

Give RhoGAM again at 72 hours postpartum to protect subsequent pregnancy

Father Rh(+)
Mother Rh(−)
AB(+)

↓

Do not administer RhoGAM
- Mother has already seen Rh(+) blood

↓

TX:
Measure antibody titers

↓

Titers ≥1:8 – perform amniocentesis

↓

Check bilirubin

Mother Rh(+)

↓

No need for RhoGAM

↓

Monitor mother and baby

OB/GYN

Vaginal Discharge 1

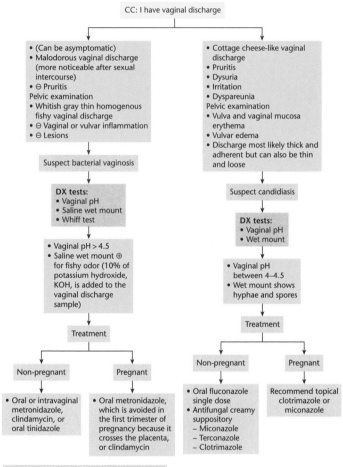

CC: I have vaginal discharge

- (Can be asymptomatic)
- Malodorous vaginal discharge (more noticeable after sexual intercourse)
- ⊖ Pruritis

Pelvic examination
- Whitish gray thin homogenous fishy vaginal discharge
- ⊖ Vaginal or vulvar inflammation
- ⊖ Lesions

Suspect bacterial vaginosis

DX tests:
- Vaginal pH
- Saline wet mount
- Whiff test

- Vaginal pH > 4.5
- Saline wet mount ⊕ for fishy odor (10% of potassium hydroxide, KOH, is added to the vaginal discharge sample)

Treatment

Non-pregnant

- Oral or intravaginal metronidazole, clindamycin, or oral tinidazole

Pregnant

- Oral metronidazole, which is avoided in the first trimester of pregnancy because it crosses the placenta, or clindamycin

Note:
- Pregnant women infected with BV are at higher risk for preterm delivery
- BV is not sexually transmitted so the patients sexual partners do not require treatment

- Cottage cheese-like vaginal discharge
- Pruritis
- Dysuria
- Irritation
- Dyspareunia

Pelvic examination
- Vulva and vaginal mucosa erythema
- Vulvar edema
- Discharge most likely thick and adherent but can also be thin and loose

Suspect candidiasis

DX tests:
- Vaginal pH
- Wet mount

- Vaginal pH between 4–4.5
- Wet mount shows hyphae and spores

Treatment

Non-pregnant

- Oral fluconazole single dose
- Antifungal creamy suppository
  – Miconazole
  – Terconazole
  – Clotrimazole

Pregnant

Recommend topical clotrimazole or miconazole

OB/GYN

Vaginal Discharge 2

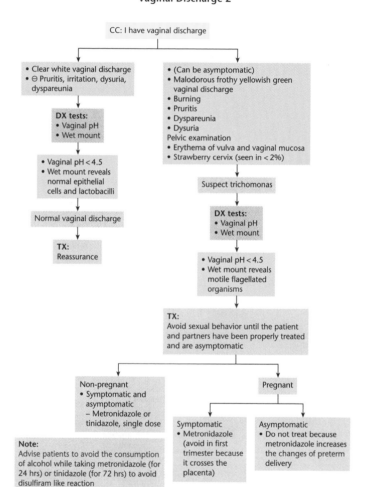

Medical Reference Guide

PEDIATRICS

Asthma

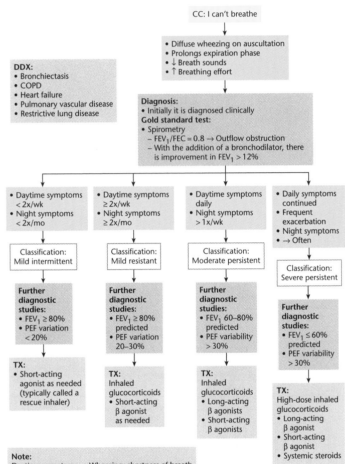

CC: I can't breathe

- Diffuse wheezing on auscultation
- Prolongs expiration phase
- ↓ Breath sounds
- ↑ Breathing effort

DDX:
- Bronchiectasis
- COPD
- Heart failure
- Pulmonary vascular disease
- Restrictive lung disease

Diagnosis:
- Initially it is diagnosed clinically

Gold standard test:
- Spirometry
  - $FEV_1/FEC = 0.8 \rightarrow$ Outflow obstruction
  - With the addition of a bronchodilator, there is improvement in $FEV_1 > 12\%$

- Daytime symptoms < 2x/wk
- Night symptoms < 2x/mo

Classification: Mild intermittent

Further diagnostic studies:
- $FEV_1 \geq 80\%$
- PEF variation < 20%

TX:
- Short-acting agonist as needed (typically called a rescue inhaler)

- Daytime symptoms ≥ 2x/wk
- Night symptoms ≥ 2x/mo

Classification: Mild resistant

Further diagnostic studies:
- $FEV_1 \geq 80\%$ predicted
- PEF variation 20–30%

TX:
Inhaled glucocorticoids
- Short-acting β agonist as needed

- Daytime symptoms daily
- Night symptoms > 1x/wk

Classification: Moderate persistent

Further diagnostic studies:
- FEV_1 60–80% predicted
- PEF variability > 30%

TX:
Inhaled glucocorticoids
- Long-acting β agonists
- Short-acting β agonists

- Daily symptoms continued
- Frequent exacerbation
- Night symptoms
- → Often

Classification: Severe persistent

Further diagnostic studies:
- $FEV_1 \leq 60\%$ predicted
- PEF variability > 30%

TX:
High-dose inhaled glucocorticoids
- Long-acting β agonist
- Short-acting β agonist
- Systemic steroids

Note:
Daytime symptoms → Wheezing, shortness of breath
Night symptoms → Awakening with cough, SOB
PEF = Peek expiratory flow

PEDIATRICS

Birth Injuries

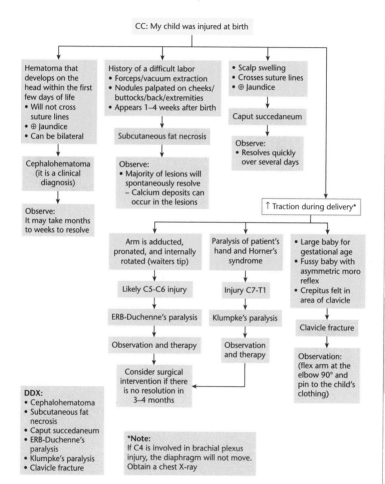

CC: My child was injured at birth

Hematoma that develops on the head within the first few days of life
• Will not cross suture lines
• ⊕ Jaundice
• Can be bilateral

↓

Cephalohematoma (it is a clinical diagnosis)

↓

Observe:
It may take months to weeks to resolve

History of a difficult labor
• Forceps/vacuum extraction
• Nodules palpated on cheeks/buttocks/back/extremities
• Appears 1–4 weeks after birth

↓

Subcutaneous fat necrosis

↓

Observe:
• Majority of lesions will spontaneously resolve
  – Calcium deposits can occur in the lesions

• Scalp swelling
• Crosses suture lines
• ⊕ Jaundice

↓

Caput succedaneum

↓

Observe:
• Resolves quickly over several days

↑ Traction during delivery*

Arm is adducted, pronated, and internally rotated (waiters tip)

↓

Likely C5-C6 injury

↓

ERB-Duchenne's paralysis

↓

Observation and therapy

↓

Consider surgical intervention if there is no resolution in 3–4 months

---

Paralysis of patient's hand and Horner's syndrome

↓

Injury C7-T1

↓

Klumpke's paralysis

↓

Observation and therapy

• Large baby for gestational age
• Fussy baby with asymmetric moro reflex
• Crepitus felt in area of clavicle

↓

Clavicle fracture

↓

Observation:
(flex arm at the elbow 90° and pin to the child's clothing)

DDX:
• Cephalohematoma
• Subcutaneous fat necrosis
• Caput succedaneum
• ERB-Duchenne's paralysis
• Klumpke's paralysis
• Clavicle fracture

*Note:
If C4 is involved in brachial plexus injury, the diaphragm will not move. Obtain a chest X-ray.

PEDIATRICS

PEDIATRICS

Cyanotic Heart Disease 1

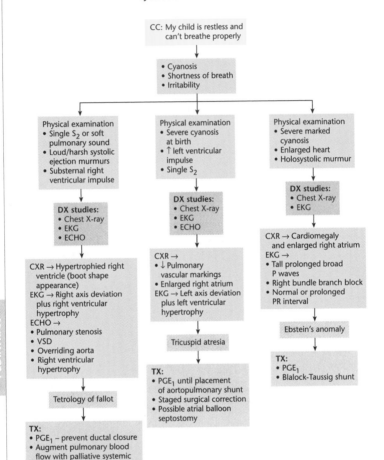

CC: My child is restless and can't breathe properly

- Cyanosis
- Shortness of breath
- Irritability

Physical examination
- Single S₂ or soft pulmonary sound
- Loud/harsh systolic ejection murmurs
- Substernal right ventricular impulse

DX studies:
- Chest X-ray
- EKG
- ECHO

CXR → Hypertrophied right ventricle (boot shape appearance)
EKG → Right axis deviation plus right ventricular hypertrophy
ECHO →
- Pulmonary stenosis
- VSD
- Overriding aorta
- Right ventricular hypertrophy

Tetrology of fallot

TX:
- PGE₁ – prevent ductal closure
- Augment pulmonary blood flow with palliative systemic to pulmonary shunt (modified Blalock-Taussig shunt)

Physical examination
- Severe cyanosis at birth
- ↑ left ventricular impulse
- Single S₂

DX studies:
- Chest X-ray
- EKG
- ECHO

CXR →
- ↓ Pulmonary vascular markings
- Enlarged right atrium
EKG → Left axis deviation plus left ventricular hypertrophy

Tricuspid atresia

TX:
- PGE₁ until placement of aortopulmonary shunt
- Staged surgical correction
- Possible atrial balloon septostomy

Physical examination
- Severe marked cyanosis
- Enlarged heart
- Holosystolic murmur

DX studies:
- Chest X-ray
- EKG

CXR → Cardiomegaly and enlarged right atrium
EKG →
- Tall prolonged broad P waves
- Right bundle branch block
- Normal or prolonged PR interval

Ebstein's anomaly

TX:
- PGE₁
- Blalock-Taussig shunt

PEDIATRICS

PEDIATRICS

Cyanotic Heart Disease 2

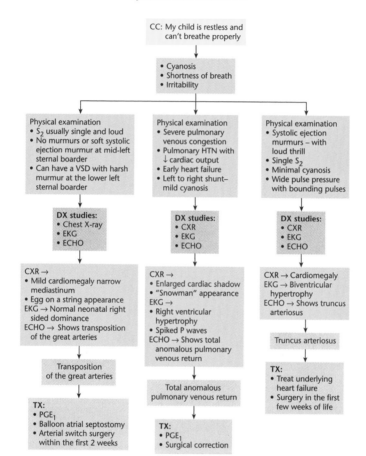

CC: My child is restless and can't breathe properly

↓

- Cyanosis
- Shortness of breath
- Irritability

Physical examination
- S_2 usually single and loud
- No murmurs or soft systolic ejection murmur at mid-left sternal boarder
- Can have a VSD with harsh murmur at the lower left sternal boarder

DX studies:
- Chest X-ray
- EKG
- ECHO

CXR →
- Mild cardiomegaly narrow mediastinum
- Egg on a string appearance
EKG → Normal neonatal right sided dominance
ECHO → Shows transposition of the great arteries

Transposition of the great arteries

TX:
- PGE_1
- Balloon atrial septostomy
- Arterial switch surgery within the first 2 weeks

Physical examination
- Severe pulmonary venous congestion
- Pulmonary HTN with ↓ cardiac output
- Early heart failure
- Left to right shunt– mild cyanosis

DX studies:
- CXR
- EKG
- ECHO

CXR →
- Enlarged cardiac shadow
- "Snowman" appearance
EKG →
- Right ventricular hypertrophy
- Spiked P waves
ECHO → Shows total anomalous pulmonary venous return

Total anomalous pulmonary venous return

TX:
- PGE_1
- Surgical correction

Physical examination
- Systolic ejection murmurs – with loud thrill
- Single S_2
- Minimal cyanosis
- Wide pulse pressure with bounding pulses

DX studies:
- CXR
- EKG
- ECHO

CXR → Cardiomegaly
EKG → Biventricular hypertrophy
ECHO → Shows truncus arteriosus

Truncus arteriosus

TX:
- Treat underlying heart failure
- Surgery in the first few weeks of life

PEDIATRICS

Development Dysplasia of Hip

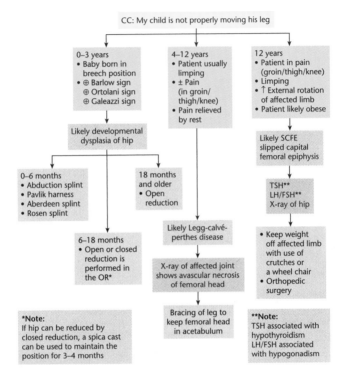

CC: My child is not properly moving his leg

0–3 years
- Baby born in breech position
- ⊕ Barlow sign
- ⊕ Ortolani sign
- ⊕ Galeazzi sign

4–12 years
- Patient usually limping
- ± Pain (in groin/thigh/knee)
- Pain relieved by rest

12 years
- Patient in pain (groin/thigh/knee)
- Limping
- ↑ External rotation of affected limb
- Patient likely obese

Likely developmental dysplasia of hip

Likely SCFE slipped capital femoral epiphysis

0–6 months
- Abduction splint
- Pavlik harness
- Aberdeen splint
- Rosen splint

18 months and older
- Open reduction

TSH**
LH/FSH**
X-ray of hip

6–18 months
- Open or closed reduction is performed in the OR*

Likely Legg-calvé-perthes disease

- Keep weight off affected limb with use of crutches or a wheel chair
- Orthopedic surgery

X-ray of affected joint shows avascular necrosis of femoral head

*Note:
If hip can be reduced by closed reduction, a spica cast can be used to maintain the position for 3–4 months

Bracing of leg to keep femoral head in acetabulum

**Note:
TSH associated with hypothyroidism
LH/FSH associated with hypogonadism

PEDIATRICS

Diarrhea

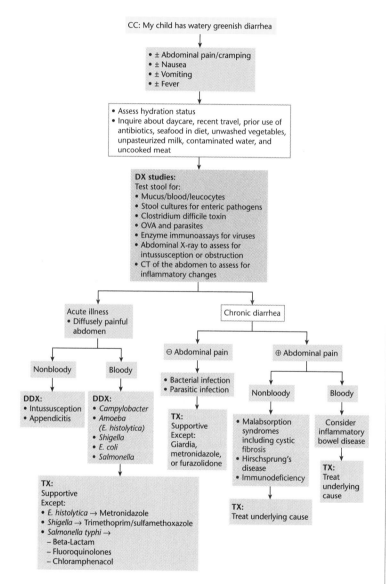

CC: My child has watery greenish diarrhea

- ± Abdominal pain/cramping
- ± Nausea
- ± Vomiting
- ± Fever

- Assess hydration status
- Inquire about daycare, recent travel, prior use of antibiotics, seafood in diet, unwashed vegetables, unpasteurized milk, contaminated water, and uncooked meat

DX studies:
Test stool for:
- Mucus/blood/leucocytes
- Stool cultures for enteric pathogens
- Clostridium difficile toxin
- OVA and parasites
- Enzyme immunoassays for viruses
- Abdominal X-ray to assess for intussusception or obstruction
- CT of the abdomen to assess for inflammatory changes

Acute illness
- Diffusely painful abdomen

Chronic diarrhea

⊖ Abdominal pain

⊕ Abdominal pain

Nonbloody

Bloody

DDX:
- Intussusception
- Appendicitis

DDX:
- Campylobacter
- Amoeba (E. histolytica)
- Shigella
- E. coli
- Salmonella

TX:
Supportive
Except:
- E. histolytica → Metronidazole
- Shigella → Trimethoprim/sulfamethoxazole
- Salmonella typhi →
  – Beta-Lactam
  – Fluoroquinolones
  – Chloramphenacol

- Bacterial infection
- Parasitic infection

TX:
Supportive
Except:
Giardia, metronidazole, or furazolidone

Nonbloody

Bloody

- Malabsorption syndromes including cystic fibrosis
- Hirschsprung's disease
- Immunodeficiency

Consider inflammatory bowel disease

TX:
Treat underlying cause

TX:
Treat underlying cause

PEDIATRICS

Diarrhea Acute/Chronic

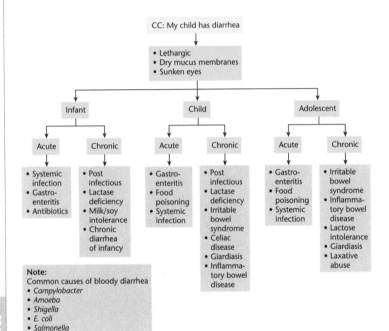

CC: My child has diarrhea

- Lethargic
- Dry mucus membranes
- Sunken eyes

Infant

Acute
- Systemic infection
- Gastro-enteritis
- Antibiotics

Chronic
- Post infectious
- Lactase deficiency
- Milk/soy intolerance
- Chronic diarrhea of infancy

Child

Acute
- Gastro-enteritis
- Food poisoning
- Systemic infection

Chronic
- Post infectious
- Lactase deficiency
- Irritable bowel syndrome
- Celiac disease
- Giardiasis
- Inflammatory bowel disease

Adolescent

Acute
- Gastro-enteritis
- Food poisoning
- Systemic infection

Chronic
- Irritable bowel syndrome
- Inflammatory bowel disease
- Lactose intolerance
- Giardiasis
- Laxative abuse

Note:
Common causes of bloody diarrhea
- *Campylobacter*
- *Amoeba*
- *Shigella*
- *E. coli*
- *Salmonella*

PEDIATRICS

Evaluation of Fever

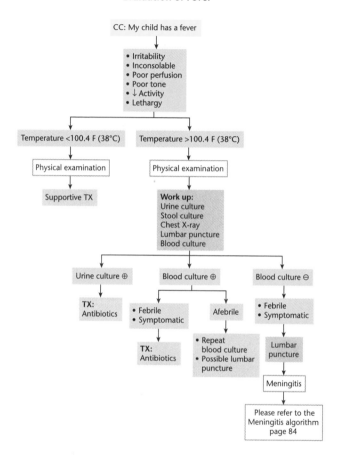

CC: My child has a fever

- Irritability
- Inconsolable
- Poor perfusion
- Poor tone
- ↓ Activity
- Lethargy

Temperature <100.4 F (38°C) → Physical examination → Supportive TX

Temperature >100.4 F (38°C) → Physical examination →

Work up:
Urine culture
Stool culture
Chest X-ray
Lumbar puncture
Blood culture

Urine culture ⊕ → **TX:** Antibiotics

Blood culture ⊕
- Febrile
- Symptomatic → **TX:** Antibiotics

Afebrile → • Repeat blood culture • Possible lumbar puncture

Blood culture ⊖
- Febrile
- Symptomatic → Lumbar puncture → Meningitis → Please refer to the Meningitis algorithm page 84

PEDIATRICS

Lead Poisoning

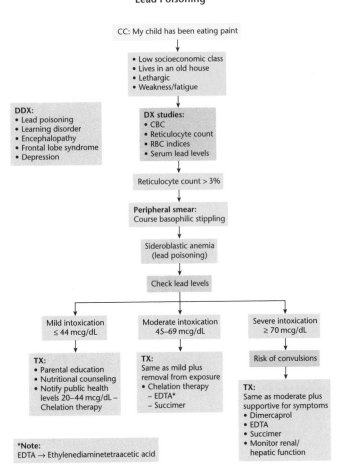

CC: My child has been eating paint

- Low socioeconomic class
- Lives in an old house
- Lethargic
- Weakness/fatigue

DDX:
- Lead poisoning
- Learning disorder
- Encephalopathy
- Frontal lobe syndrome
- Depression

DX studies:
- CBC
- Reticulocyte count
- RBC indices
- Serum lead levels

Reticulocyte count > 3%

Peripheral smear:
Course basophilic stippling

Sideroblastic anemia
(lead poisoning)

Check lead levels

Mild intoxication
≤ 44 mcg/dL

Moderate intoxication
45–69 mcg/dL

Severe intoxication
≥ 70 mcg/dL

TX:
- Parental education
- Nutritional counseling
- Notify public health
  levels 20–44 mcg/dL –
  Chelation therapy

TX:
Same as mild plus
removal from exposure
- Chelation therapy
  – EDTA*
  – Succimer

Risk of convulsions

TX:
Same as moderate plus
supportive for symptoms
- Dimercaprol
- EDTA
- Succimer
- Monitor renal/
  hepatic function

*Note:
EDTA → Ethylenediaminetetraacetic acid

PEDIATRICS

Left to Right Shunt

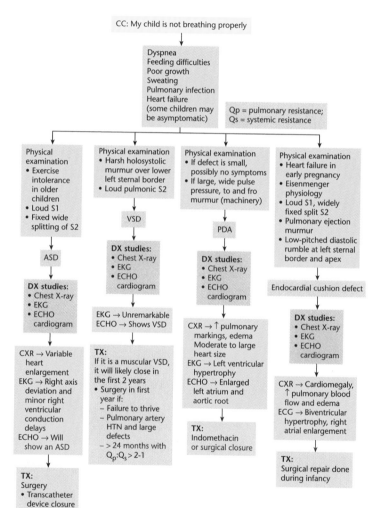

CC: My child is not breathing properly

Dyspnea
Feeding difficulties
Poor growth
Sweating
Pulmonary infection
Heart failure
(some children may
be asymptomatic)

Qp = pulmonary resistance;
Qs = systemic resistance

Physical examination
• Exercise intolerance in older children
• Loud S1
• Fixed wide splitting of S2

ASD

DX studies:
• Chest X-ray
• EKG
• ECHO cardiogram

CXR → Variable heart enlargement
EKG → Right axis deviation and minor right ventricular conduction delays
ECHO → Will show an ASD

TX:
Surgery
• Transcatheter device closure

Physical examination
• Harsh holosystolic murmur over lower left sternal border
• Loud pulmonic S2

VSD

DX studies:
• Chest X-ray
• EKG
• ECHO cardiogram

EKG → Unremarkable
ECHO → Shows VSD

TX:
If it is a muscular VSD, it will likely close in the first 2 years
• Surgery in first year if:
  – Failure to thrive
  – Pulmonary artery HTN and large defects
  – > 24 months with $Q_p:Q_s > 2\text{-}1$

Physical examination
• If defect is small, possibly no symptoms
• If large, wide pulse pressure, to and fro murmur (machinery)

PDA

DX studies:
• Chest X-ray
• EKG
• ECHO cardiogram

CXR → ↑ pulmonary markings, edema Moderate to large heart size
EKG → Left ventricular hypertrophy
ECHO → Enlarged left atrium and aortic root

TX:
Indomethacin or surgical closure

Physical examination
• Heart failure in early pregnancy
• Eisenmenger physiology
• Loud S1, widely fixed split S2
• Pulmonary ejection murmur
• Low-pitched diastolic rumble at left sternal border and apex

Endocardial cushion defect

DX studies:
• Chest X-ray
• EKG
• ECHO cardiogram

CXR → Cardiomegaly, ↑ pulmonary blood flow and edema
ECG → Biventricular hypertrophy, right atrial enlargement

TX:
Surgical repair done during infancy

PEDIATRICS

PEDIATRICS
Meningitis

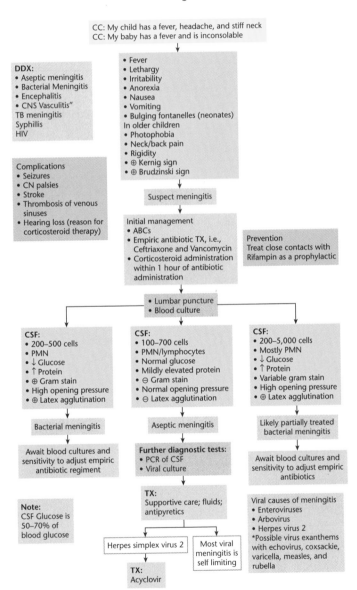

CC: My child has a fever, headache, and stiff neck
CC: My baby has a fever and is inconsolable

DDX:
- Aseptic meningitis
- Bacterial Meningitis
- Encephalitis
- CNS Vasculitis"
TB meningitis
Syphillis
HIV

• Fever
• Lethargy
• Irritability
• Anorexia
• Nausea
• Vomiting
• Bulging fontanelles (neonates)
In older children
• Photophobia
• Neck/back pain
• Rigidity
• ⊕ Kernig sign
• ⊕ Brudzinski sign

Complications
• Seizures
• CN palsies
• Stroke
• Thrombosis of venous sinuses
• Hearing loss (reason for corticosteroid therapy)

Suspect meningitis

Initial management
• ABCs
• Empiric antibiotic TX, i.e., Ceftriaxone and Vancomycin
• Corticosteroid administration within 1 hour of antibiotic administration

Prevention
Treat close contacts with Rifampin as a prophylactic

• Lumbar puncture
• Blood culture

CSF:
• 200–500 cells
• PMN
• ↓ Glucose
• ↑ Protein
• ⊕ Gram stain
• High opening pressure
• ⊕ Latex agglutination

CSF:
• 100–700 cells
• PMN/lymphocytes
• Normal glucose
• Mildly elevated protein
• ⊖ Gram stain
• Normal opening pressure
• ⊖ Latex agglutination

CSF:
• 200–5,000 cells
• Mostly PMN
• ↓ Glucose
• ↑ Protein
• Variable gram stain
• High opening pressure
• ⊕ Latex agglutination

Bacterial meningitis

Aseptic meningitis

Likely partially treated bacterial meningitis

Await blood cultures and sensitivity to adjust empiric antibiotic regimen

Further diagnostic tests:
• PCR of CSF
• Viral culture

Await blood cultures and sensitivity to adjust empiric antibiotics

Note:
CSF Glucose is 50–70% of blood glucose

TX:
Supportive care; fluids; antipyretics

Viral causes of meningitis
• Enteroviruses
• Arbovirus
• Herpes virus 2
*Possible virus exanthems with echovirus, coxsackie, varicella, measles, and rubella

Herpes simplex virus 2

Most viral meningitis is self limiting

TX:
Acyclovir

Algorithms

PEDIATRICS

Myocardial Disease

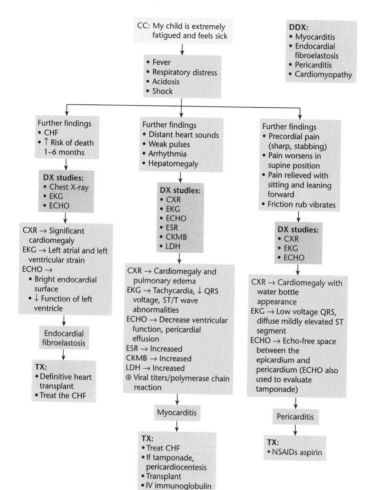

CC: My child is extremely fatigued and feels sick

DDX:
- Myocarditis
- Endocardial fibroelastosis
- Pericarditis
- Cardiomyopathy

- Fever
- Respiratory distress
- Acidosis
- Shock

Further findings
- CHF
- ↑ Risk of death 1–6 months

DX studies:
- Chest X-ray
- EKG
- ECHO

CXR → Significant cardiomegaly
EKG → Left atrial and left ventricular strain
ECHO →
- Bright endocardial surface
- ↓ Function of left ventricle

Endocardial fibroelastosis

TX:
- Definitive heart transplant
- Treat the CHF

Further findings
- Distant heart sounds
- Weak pulses
- Arrhythmia
- Hepatomegaly

DX studies:
- CXR
- EKG
- ECHO
- ESR
- CKMB
- LDH

CXR → Cardiomegaly and pulmonary edema
EKG → Tachycardia, ↓ QRS voltage, ST/T wave abnormalities
ECHO → Decrease ventricular function, pericardial effusion
ESR → Increased
CKMB → Increased
LDH → Increased
⊕ Viral titers/polymerase chain reaction

Myocarditis

TX:
- Treat CHF
- If tamponade, pericardiocentesis
- Transplant
- IV immunoglobulin

Further findings
- Precordial pain (sharp, stabbing)
- Pain worsens in supine position
- Pain relieved with sitting and leaning forward
- Friction rub vibrates

DX studies:
- CXR
- EKG
- ECHO

CXR → Cardiomegaly with water bottle appearance
EKG → Low voltage QRS, diffuse mildly elevated ST segment
ECHO → Echo-free space between the epicardium and pericardium (ECHO also used to evaluate tamponade)

Pericarditis

TX:
- NSAIDs aspirin

PEDIATRICS

PEDIATRICS

Otitis

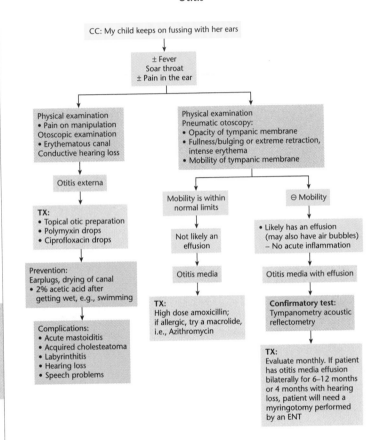

CC: My child keeps on fussing with her ears

± Fever
Soar throat
± Pain in the ear

Physical examination
• Pain on manipulation
Otoscopic examination
• Erythematous canal
Conductive hearing loss

Otitis externa

TX:
• Topical otic preparation
• Polymyxin drops
• Ciprofloxacin drops

Prevention:
Earplugs, drying of canal
• 2% acetic acid after
getting wet, e.g., swimming

Complications:
• Acute mastoiditis
• Acquired cholesteatoma
• Labyrinthitis
• Hearing loss
• Speech problems

Physical examination
Pneumatic otoscopy:
• Opacity of tympanic membrane
• Fullness/bulging or extreme retraction,
intense erythema
• Mobility of tympanic membrane

Mobility is within
normal limits

⊖ Mobility

Not likely an
effusion

• Likely has an effusion
(may also have air bubbles)
– No acute inflammation

Otitis media

Otitis media with effusion

TX:
High dose amoxicillin;
if allergic, try a macrolide,
i.e., Azithromycin

Confirmatory test:
Tympanometry acoustic
reflectometry

TX:
Evaluate monthly. If patient
has otitis media effusion
bilaterally for 6–12 months
or 4 months with hearing
loss, patient will need a
myringotomy performed
by an ENT

PEDIATRICS

Pharyngitis

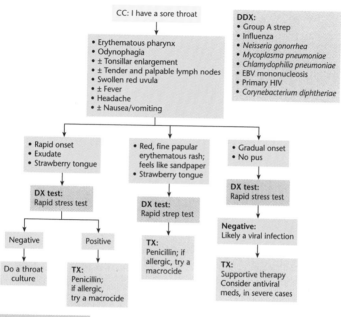

CC: I have a sore throat

DDX:
- Group A strep
- Influenza
- *Neisseria gonorrhea*
- *Mycoplasma pneumoniae*
- *Chlamydophilia pneumoniae*
- EBV mononucleosis
- Primary HIV
- *Corynebacterium diphtheriae*

- Erythematous pharynx
- Odynophagia
- ± Tonsillar enlargement
- ± Tender and palpable lymph nodes
- Swollen red uvula
- ± Fever
- Headache
- ± Nausea/vomiting

- Rapid onset
- Exudate
- Strawberry tongue

- Red, fine papular erythematous rash; feels like sandpaper
- Strawberry tongue

- Gradual onset
- No pus

DX test:
Rapid stress test

DX test:
Rapid strep test

DX test:
Rapid stress test

Negative

Positive

TX:
Penicillin; if allergic, try a macrocide

Negative:
Likely a viral infection

Do a throat culture

TX:
Penicillin; if allergic, try a macrocide

TX:
Supportive therapy
Consider antiviral meds, in severe cases

Complications
- Retropharyngeal/lateral pharyngeal abscess
- Peritonsillar abscess

Note:
Indications for tonsillectomy
Rate of strep throat
   5 infections/year for 2 years
   3 infections/year for 3 years
Indications for adenoidectomy
- Nasal obstruction → Persistent symptoms
- Refractory chronic sinusitis
- Recurrent otitis media/chronic otitis media with effusion with tympanoscopy tubes that have been removed

PEDIATRICS

Pnuemonia

CC: My child has a fever and cough

- ⊕ Fever (May be as high as 40°C (104°F))
- Tachypnea
- ⊕ Productive cough
- ⊕ Chest pain
- ⊕ Dehydration
- ⊕ Inability to feed

Complications
Pleural effusion
Empyema
Lung abscess
Pneumatocele
Necrotizing pneumonia
Hyponatremia

DDX:
- Respiratory distress syndrome
- Atelectasis
- Bronchiolitis
- Acute exacerbation of asthma

- CBC (will have ↑↑ WBC)
- Blood culture
- Chest X-ray
- Nasopharyngeal washing (to detect RSV)
- Lung auscultation (↓ breath sounds, scattering crackles, dullness to percussion)

CXR:
Hyperinflation with bilateral interstitial infiltrates; peribronchial cuffing

CXR: Confluent lobar consolidation

- WBCs 15,000–40,000/mm^3
- Sudden shaking chills
- High fever

- WBCs may not be elevated
- WBCs < 20,000/mm^3 with lymphocyte predominance

Likely bacterial

Likely viral

Nosocomial infection

Aspiration pneumonia

If mild, no respiratory distress

If severe, ⊕ respiratory distress

- Develops during hospitalization
- Develops after a recent hospitalization

TX:
Treats as if it were community acquired pneumonia, plus cover for anaerobes ampicillin-sulbactam or clindamycin
- If aspiration occurred during hospitalization, tx as nosocomial pneumonia

TX:
- Supportive
- Fluids
- Antipyretics

Consider:
Staphylococcus aureus, pseudomonas, anaerobes, enterobacteriaceae

⊖ RSV

⊕ RSV

TX:
Broad spectrum empiric antibiotics + aminoglycosides
- Ticarcillin-clavulanate piperacillin-tazobactam meropenen

***Note:**
If resistant, use culture and sensitivity
- Sputum culture not of much value in children

Suspect co-infection with bacteria

TX:
Ribavirin
± Corticosteriods
± RSV immunoglobulins

If allergic to beta-lactam, use clindamycin

1

Continued on Next Page

PEDIATRICS

PEDIATRICS

Pnuemonia *(continued)*

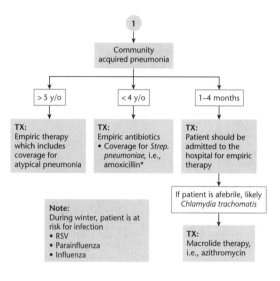

1

Community acquired pneumonia

> 5 y/o

TX:
Empiric therapy which includes coverage for atypical pneumonia

< 4 y/o

TX:
Empiric antibiotics
• Coverage for *Strep. pneumoniae*, i.e., amoxicillin*

Note:
During winter, patient is at risk for infection
• RSV
• Parainfluenza
• Influenza

1–4 months

TX:
Patient should be admitted to the hospital for empiric therapy

If patient is afebrile, likely *Chlamydia trachomatis*

TX:
Macrolide therapy, i.e., azithromycin

PEDIATRICS
Red Eye

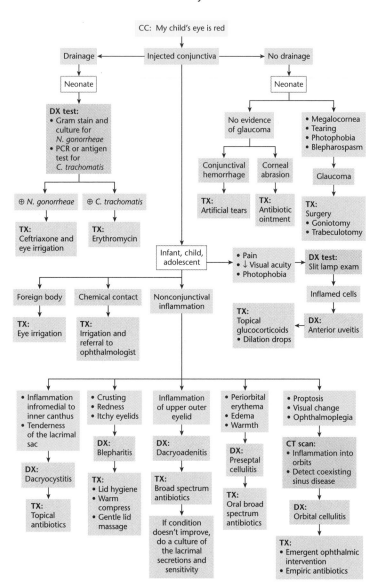

PEDIATRICS

Respiratory Distress in a Child

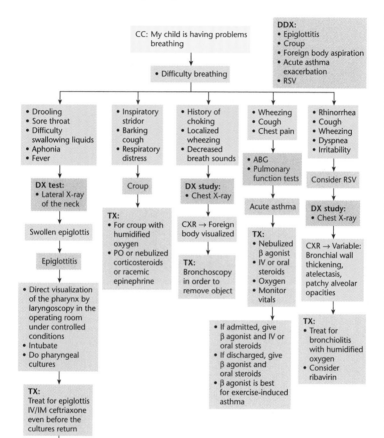

CC: My child is having problems breathing

DDX:
- Epiglottitis
- Croup
- Foreign body aspiration
- Acute asthma exacerbation
- RSV

• Difficulty breathing

Branch 1:
- Drooling
- Sore throat
- Difficulty swallowing liquids
- Aphonia
- Fever

DX test:
- Lateral X-ray of the neck

Swollen epiglottis

Epiglottitis

- Direct visualization of the pharynx by laryngoscopy in the operating room under controlled conditions
- Intubate
- Do pharyngeal cultures

TX:
Treat for epiglottis IV/IM ceftriaxone even before the cultures return

- Artificial airway
- Supplemental oxygen

Branch 2:
- Inspiratory stridor
- Barking cough
- Respiratory distress

Croup

TX:
- For croup with humidified oxygen
- PO or nebulized corticosteroids or racemic epinephrine

Branch 3:
- History of choking
- Localized wheezing
- Decreased breath sounds

DX study:
- Chest X-ray

CXR → Foreign body visualized

TX:
Bronchoscopy in order to remove object

Branch 4:
- Wheezing
- Cough
- Chest pain

- ABG
- Pulmonary function tests

Acute asthma

TX:
- Nebulized β agonist
- IV or oral steroids
- Oxygen
- Monitor vitals

- If admitted, give β agonist and IV or oral steroids
- If discharged, give β agonist and oral steroids
- β agonist is best for exercise-induced asthma

Branch 5:
- Rhinorrhea
- Cough
- Wheezing
- Dyspnea
- Irritability

Consider RSV

DX study:
- Chest X-ray

CXR → Variable: Bronchial wall thickening, atelectasis, patchy alveolar opacities

TX:
- Treat for bronchiolitis with humidified oxygen
- Consider ribavirin

PEDIATRICS

Salmon Patch/Capillary Hemangioma/Nevus Sebaceous

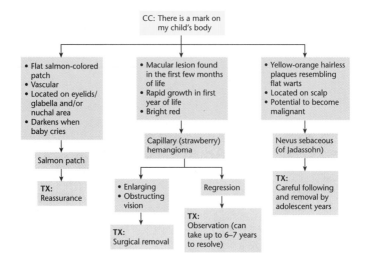

CC: There is a mark on my child's body

• Flat salmon-colored patch
• Vascular
• Located on eyelids/glabella and/or nuchal area
• Darkens when baby cries

↓

Salmon patch

↓

TX: Reassurance

• Macular lesion found in the first few months of life
• Rapid growth in first year of life
• Bright red

↓

Capillary (strawberry) hemangioma

• Enlarging
• Obstructing vision

TX: Surgical removal

Regression

TX: Observation (can take up to 6–7 years to resolve)

• Yellow-orange hairless plaques resembling flat warts
• Located on scalp
• Potential to become malignant

↓

Nevus sebaceous (of Jadassohn)

↓

TX: Careful following and removal by adolescent years

Scoliosis

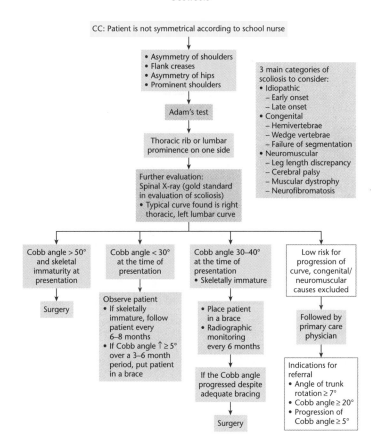

CC: Patient is not symmetrical according to school nurse

- Asymmetry of shoulders
- Flank creases
- Asymmetry of hips
- Prominent shoulders

3 main categories of scoliosis to consider:
- Idiopathic
  - Early onset
  - Late onset
- Congenital
  - Hemivertebrae
  - Wedge vertebrae
  - Failure of segmentation
- Neuromuscular
  - Leg length discrepancy
  - Cerebral palsy
  - Muscular dystrophy
  - Neurofibromatosis

Adam's test

Thoracic rib or lumbar prominence on one side

Further evaluation:
Spinal X-ray (gold standard in evaluation of scoliosis)
- Typical curve found is right thoracic, left lumbar curve

Cobb angle > 50° and skeletal immaturity at presentation → Surgery

Cobb angle < 30° at the time of presentation → Observe patient
- If skeletally immature, follow patient every 6–8 months
- If Cobb angle ↑ ≥ 5° over a 3–6 month period, put patient in a brace

Cobb angle 30–40° at the time of presentation
- Skeletally immature
- Place patient in a brace
- Radiographic monitoring every 6 months

If the Cobb angle progressed despite adequate bracing → Surgery

Low risk for progression of curve, congenital/neuromuscular causes excluded → Followed by primary care physician

Indications for referral
- Angle of trunk rotation ≥ 7°
- Cobb angle ≥ 20°
- Progression of Cobb angle ≥ 5°

PEDIATRICS

PEDIATRICS

Viral Exanthems

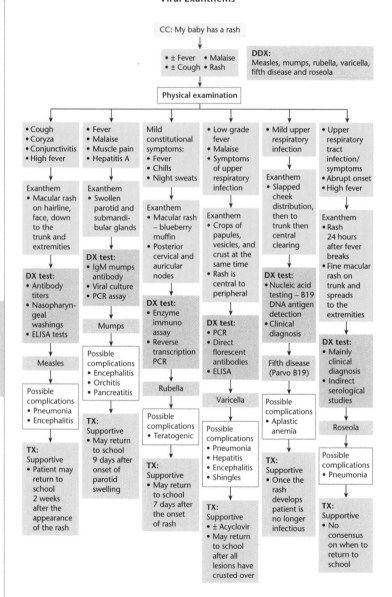

CC: My baby has a rash

- ± Fever
- ± Cough
- Malaise
- Rash

DDX:
Measles, mumps, rubella, varicella, fifth disease and roseola

Physical examination

- Cough
- Coryza
- Conjunctivitis
- High fever

Exanthem
- Macular rash on hairline, face, down to the trunk and extremities

DX test:
- Antibody titers
- Nasopharyngeal washings
- ELISA tests

Measles

Possible complications
- Pneumonia
- Encephalitis

TX:
Supportive
- Patient may return to school 2 weeks after the appearance of the rash

---

- Fever
- Malaise
- Muscle pain
- Hepatitis A

Exanthem
- Swollen parotid and submandibular glands

DX test:
- IgM mumps antibody
- Viral culture
- PCR assay

Mumps

Possible complications
- Encephalitis
- Orchitis
- Pancreatitis

TX:
Supportive
- May return to school 9 days after onset of parotid swelling

---

Mild constitutional symptoms:
- Fever
- Chills
- Night sweats

Exanthem
- Macular rash – blueberry muffin
- Posterior cervical and auricular nodes

DX test:
- Enzyme immuno assay
- Reverse transcription PCR

Rubella

Possible complications
- Teratogenic

TX:
Supportive
- May return to school 7 days after the onset of rash

- Low grade fever
- Malaise
- Symptoms of upper respiratory infection

Exanthem
- Crops of papules, vesicles, and crust at the same time
- Rash is central to peripheral

DX test:
- PCR
- Direct florescent antibodies
- ELISA

Varicella

Possible complications
- Pneumonia
- Hepatitis
- Encephalitis
- Shingles

TX:
Supportive
- ± Acyclovir
- May return to school after all lesions have crusted over

- Mild upper respiratory infection

Exanthem
- Slapped cheek distribution, then to trunk then central clearing

DX test:
- Nucleic acid testing – B19 DNA antigen detection
- Clinical diagnosis

Fifth disease (Parvo B19)

Possible complications
- Aplastic anemia

TX:
Supportive
- Once the rash develops patient is no longer infectious

- Upper respiratory tract infection/ symptoms
- Abrupt onset
- High fever

Exanthem
- Rash 24 hours after fever breaks
- Fine macular rash on trunk and spreads to the extremities

DX test:
- Mainly clinical diagnosis
- Indirect serological studies

Roseola

Possible complications
- Pneumonia

TX:
Supportive
- No consensus on when to return to school

SURGERY

Abdominal Aortic Aneurysm

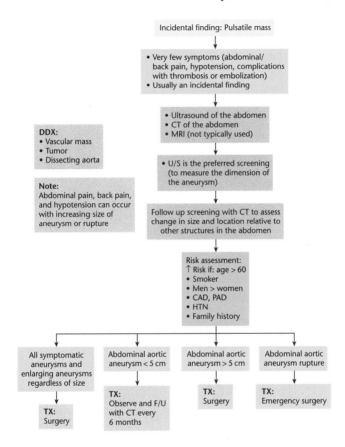

Incidental finding: Pulsatile mass

- Very few symptoms (abdominal/
  back pain, hypotension, complications
  with thrombosis or embolization)
- Usually an incidental finding

- Ultrasound of the abdomen
- CT of the abdomen
- MRI (not typically used)

- U/S is the preferred screening
  (to measure the dimension of
  the aneurysm)

Follow up screening with CT to assess
change in size and location relative to
other structures in the abdomen

Risk assessment:
↑ Risk if: age > 60
- Smoker
- Men > women
- CAD, PAD
- HTN
- Family history

DDX:
- Vascular mass
- Tumor
- Dissecting aorta

Note:
Abdominal pain, back pain,
and hypotension can occur
with increasing size of
aneurysm or rupture

All symptomatic
aneurysms and
enlarging aneurysms
regardless of size

TX:
Surgery

Abdominal aortic
aneurysm < 5 cm

TX:
Observe and F/U
with CT every
6 months

Abdominal aortic
aneurysm > 5 cm

TX:
Surgery

Abdominal aortic
aneurysm rupture

TX:
Emergency surgery

SURGERY

Medical Reference Guide

SURGERY

Abdominal Trauma

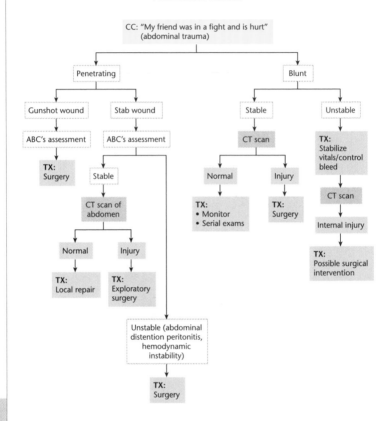

SURGERY

SURGERY

Acute Mesenteric Ischemia

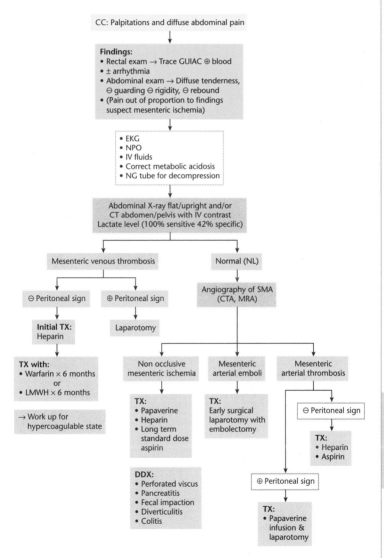

CC: Palpitations and diffuse abdominal pain

Findings:
- Rectal exam → Trace GUIAC ⊕ blood
- ± arrhythmia
- Abdominal exam → Diffuse tenderness, ⊖ guarding ⊖ rigidity, ⊖ rebound
- (Pain out of proportion to findings suspect mesenteric ischemia)

- EKG
- NPO
- IV fluids
- Correct metabolic acidosis
- NG tube for decompression

Abdominal X-ray flat/upright and/or CT abdomen/pelvis with IV contrast
Lactate level (100% sensitive 42% specific)

Mesenteric venous thrombosis

⊖ Peritoneal sign

Initial TX: Heparin

TX with:
- Warfarin × 6 months
  or
- LMWH × 6 months

→ Work up for hypercoagulable state

⊕ Peritoneal sign

Laparotomy

Normal (NL)

Angiography of SMA (CTA, MRA)

Non occlusive mesenteric ischemia

TX:
- Papaverine
- Heparin
- Long term standard dose aspirin

DDX:
- Perforated viscus
- Pancreatitis
- Fecal impaction
- Diverticulitis
- Colitis

Mesenteric arterial emboli

TX: Early surgical laparotomy with embolectomy

Mesenteric arterial thrombosis

⊖ Peritoneal sign

TX:
- Heparin
- Aspirin

⊕ Peritoneal sign

TX:
- Papaverine infusion & laparotomy

SURGERY

SURGERY

Appendicitis

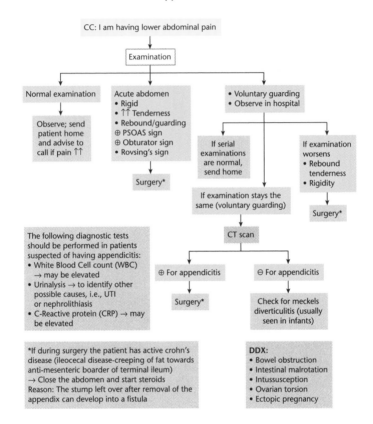

CC: I am having lower abdominal pain

Examination

Normal examination

Observe; send patient home and advise to call if pain ↑↑

Acute abdomen
- Rigid
- ↑↑ Tenderness
- Rebound/guarding
- ⊕ PSOAS sign
- ⊕ Obturator sign
- Rovsing's sign

Surgery*

- Voluntary guarding
- Observe in hospital

If serial examinations are normal, send home

If examination stays the same (voluntary guarding)

If examination worsens
- Rebound tenderness
- Rigidity

Surgery*

CT scan

⊕ For appendicitis

Surgery*

⊖ For appendicitis

Check for meckels diverticulitis (usually seen in infants)

The following diagnostic tests should be performed in patients suspected of having appendicitis:
- White Blood Cell count (WBC) → may be elevated
- Urinalysis → to identify other possible causes, i.e., UTI or nephrolithiasis
- C-Reactive protein (CRP) → may be elevated

*If during surgery the patient has active crohn's disease (ileocecal disease-creeping of fat towards anti-mesenteric boarder of terminal ileum) → Close the abdomen and start steroids
Reason: The stump left over after removal of the appendix can develop into a fistula

DDX:
- Bowel obstruction
- Intestinal malrotation
- Intussusception
- Ovarian torsion
- Ectopic pregnancy

SURGERY

Arterial Embolus

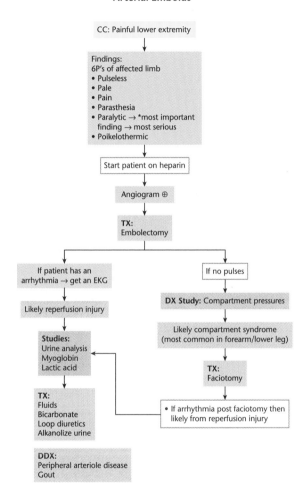

CC: Painful lower extremity

Findings:
6P's of affected limb
• Pulseless
• Pale
• Pain
• Parasthesia
• Paralytic → *most important finding → most serious
• Poikelothermic

Start patient on heparin

Angiogram ⊕

TX:
Embolectomy

If patient has an arrhythmia → get an EKG

Likely reperfusion injury

Studies:
Urine analysis
Myoglobin
Lactic acid

TX:
Fluids
Bicarbonate
Loop diuretics
Alkanolize urine

DDX:
Peripheral arteriole disease
Gout

If no pulses

DX Study: Compartment pressures

Likely compartment syndrome
(most common in forearm/lower leg)

TX:
Faciotomy

• If arrhythmia post faciotomy then likely from reperfusion injury

Medical Reference Guide

Cholangitis

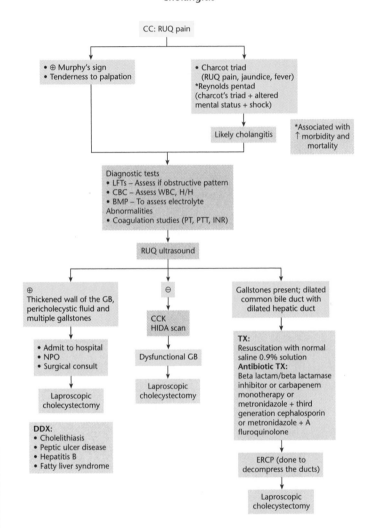

SURGERY

Diabetic Foot Ulcer

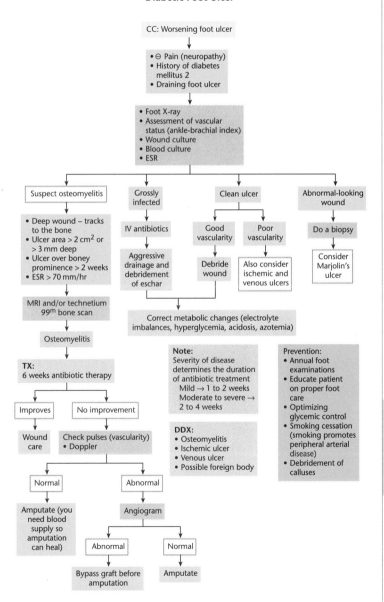

SURGERY
Esophageal Perforation

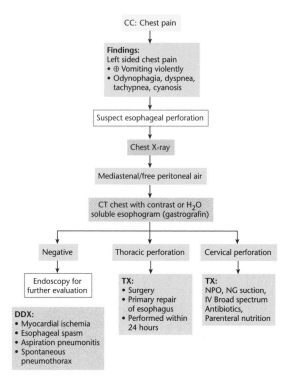

CC: Chest pain

Findings:
Left sided chest pain
• ⊕ Vomiting violently
• Odynophagia, dyspnea,
  tachypnea, cyanosis

Suspect esophageal perforation

Chest X-ray

Mediastenal/free peritoneal air

CT chest with contrast or H_2O
soluble esophogram (gastrografin)

Negative

Thoracic perforation

Cervical perforation

Endoscopy for
further evaluation

TX:
• Surgery
• Primary repair
  of esophagus
• Performed within
  24 hours

TX:
NPO, NG suction,
IV Broad spectrum
Antibiotics,
Parenteral nutrition

DDX:
• Myocardial ischemia
• Esophageal spasm
• Aspiration pneumonitis
• Spontaneous
  pneumothorax

SURGERY

Pneumothorax

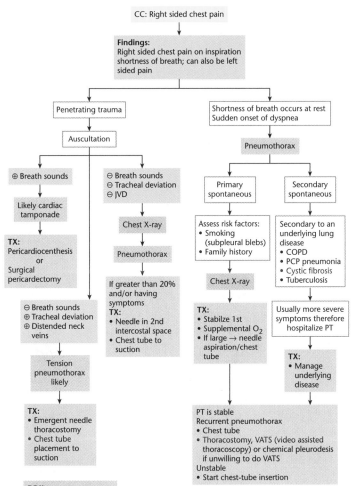

CC: Right sided chest pain

Findings:
Right sided chest pain on inspiration shortness of breath; can also be left sided pain

Penetrating trauma

Auscultation

⊕ Breath sounds

Likely cardiac tamponade

TX:
Pericardiocenthesis
or
Surgical pericardectomy

⊖ Breath sounds
⊕ Tracheal deviation
⊕ Distended neck veins

Tension pneumothorax likely

TX:
• Emergent needle thoracostomy
• Chest tube placement to suction

DDX:
• Esophageal spasm
• Myocardial ischemia
• Acute pericarditis
• Pleurodynia
• Pulmonary embolism
• Pneumothorax
• Tension pneumothorax
• Cardiac tamponade

⊖ Breath sounds
⊖ Tracheal deviation
⊖ JVD

Chest X-ray

Pneumothorax

If greater than 20% and/or having symptoms
TX:
• Needle in 2nd intercostal space
• Chest tube to suction

Shortness of breath occurs at rest
Sudden onset of dyspnea

Pneumothorax

Primary spontaneous

Assess risk factors:
• Smoking (subpleural blebs)
• Family history

Chest X-ray

TX:
• Stabilze 1st
• Supplemental O_2
• If large → needle aspiration/chest tube

Secondary spontaneous

Secondary to an underlying lung disease
• COPD
• PCP pneumonia
• Cystic fibrosis
• Tuberculosis

Usually more severe symptoms therefore hospitalize PT

TX:
• Manage underlying disease

PT is stable
Recurrent pneumothorax
• Chest tube
• Thoracostomy, VATS (video assisted thoracoscopy) or chemical pleurodesis if unwilling to do VATS
Unstable
• Start chest-tube insertion

SURGERY
Small Bowel Obstruction/Volvulus/Ogilvie Syndrome

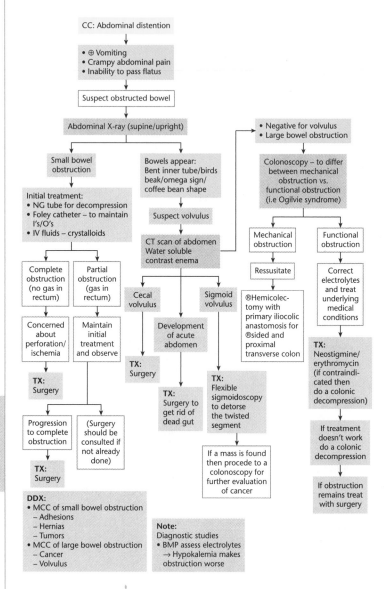

CC: Abdominal distention

- ⊕ Vomiting
- Crampy abdominal pain
- Inability to pass flatus

Suspect obstructed bowel

Abdominal X-ray (supine/upright)

Small bowel obstruction

- Negative for volvulus
- Large bowel obstruction

Bowels appear:
Bent inner tube/birds beak/omega sign/coffee bean shape

Colonoscopy – to differ between mechanical obstruction vs. functional obstruction (i.e Ogilvie syndrome)

Initial treatment:
- NG tube for decompression
- Foley catheter – to maintain I's/O's
- IV fluids – crystalloids

Suspect volvulus

CT scan of abdomen Water soluble contrast enema

Mechanical obstruction

Functional obstruction

Complete obstruction (no gas in rectum)

Partial obstruction (gas in rectum)

Cecal volvulus

Sigmoid volvulus

Ressusitate

Correct electrolytes and treat underlying medical conditions

Concerned about perforation/ ischemia

Maintain initial treatment and observe

Development of acute abdomen

®Hemicolectomy with primary iliocolic anastomosis for ®sided and proximal transverse colon

TX: Surgery

TX: Surgery

TX: Neostigmine/ erythromycin (if contraindicated then do a colonic decompression)

Progression to complete obstruction

(Surgery should be consulted if not already done)

TX: Surgery to get rid of dead gut

TX: Flexible sigmoidoscopy to detorse the twisted segment

TX: Surgery

If a mass is found then procede to a colonoscopy for further evaluation of cancer

If treatment doesn't work do a colonic decompression

If obstruction remains treat with surgery

DDX:
- MCC of small bowel obstruction
  – Adhesions
  – Hernias
  – Tumors
- MCC of large bowel obstruction
  – Cancer
  – Volvulus

Note:
Diagnostic studies
- BMP assess electrolytes → Hypokalemia makes obstruction worse

SURGERY

Testicular Torsion

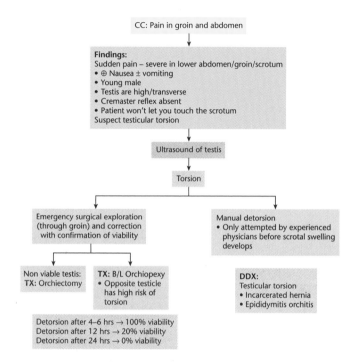

CC: Pain in groin and abdomen

Findings:
Sudden pain – severe in lower abdomen/groin/scrotum
- ⊕ Nausea ± vomiting
- Young male
- Testis are high/transverse
- Cremaster reflex absent
- Patient won't let you touch the scrotum
Suspect testicular torsion

Ultrasound of testis

Torsion

Emergency surgical exploration (through groin) and correction with confirmation of viability

Manual detorsion
- Only attempted by experienced physicians before scrotal swelling develops

Non viable testis: **TX:** Orchiectomy

TX: B/L Orchiopexy
- Opposite testicle has high risk of torsion

DDX:
Testicular torsion
- Incarcerated hernia
- Epididymitis orchitis

Detorsion after 4–6 hrs → 100% viability
Detorsion after 12 hrs → 20% viability
Detorsion after 24 hrs → 0% viability

SURGERY

Thyroid Nodule

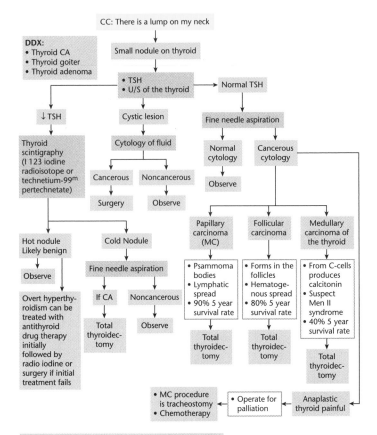

CC: There is a lump on my neck

DDX:
• Thyroid CA
• Thyroid goiter
• Thyroid adenoma

Small nodule on thyroid

• TSH
• U/S of the thyroid → Normal TSH

↓ TSH

Cystic lesion

Fine needle aspiration

Thyroid scintigraphy (I 123 iodine radioisotope or technetium-99ᵐ pertechnetate)

Cytology of fluid

Normal cytology → Observe

Cancerous cytology

Cancerous → Surgery

Noncancerous → Observe

Hot nodule Likely benign → Observe

Cold Nodule

Papillary carcinoma (MC)

Follicular carcinoma

Medullary carcinoma of the thyroid

Overt hyperthyroidism can be treated with antithyroid drug therapy initially followed by radio iodine or surgery if initial treatment fails

Fine needle aspiration

If CA → Total thyroidectomy

Noncancerous → Observe

• Psammoma bodies
• Lymphatic spread
• 90% 5 year survival rate
→ Total thyroidectomy

• Forms in the follicles
• Hematogenous spread
• 80% 5 year survival rate
→ Total thyroidectomy

• From C-cells produces calcitonin
• Suspect Men II syndrome
• 40% 5 year survival rate
→ Total thyroidectomy

• MC procedure is tracheostomy
• Chemotherapy ← • Operate for palliation ← Anaplastic thyroid painful

Note:
Worst prognostic factor for thyroid CA is capsular invasion
Complications of thyroid surgery:
• Recurrent laryngeal nerve injury
  – Unilateral → Hoarseness
  – Bilateral → Would have to perform tracheostomy
• Hypoparathyroidism

PSYCHIATRY

Bipolar Disorder

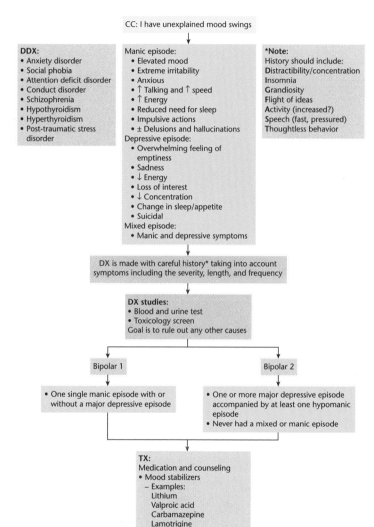

CC: I have unexplained mood swings

DDX:
- Anxiety disorder
- Social phobia
- Attention deficit disorder
- Conduct disorder
- Schizophrenia
- Hypothyroidism
- Hyperthyroidism
- Post-traumatic stress disorder

Manic episode:
- Elevated mood
- Extreme irritability
- Anxious
- ↑ Talking and ↑ speed
- ↑ Energy
- Reduced need for sleep
- Impulsive actions
- ± Delusions and hallucinations

Depressive episode:
- Overwhelming feeling of emptiness
- Sadness
- ↓ Energy
- Loss of interest
- ↓ Concentration
- Change in sleep/appetite
- Suicidal

Mixed episode:
- Manic and depressive symptoms

*Note:
History should include:
Distractibility/concentration
Insomnia
Grandiosity
Flight of ideas
Activity (increased?)
Speech (fast, pressured)
Thoughtless behavior

DX is made with careful history* taking into account symptoms including the severity, length, and frequency

DX studies:
- Blood and urine test
- Toxicology screen
Goal is to rule out any other causes

Bipolar 1
- One single manic episode with or without a major depressive episode

Bipolar 2
- One or more major depressive episode accompanied by at least one hypomanic episode
- Never had a mixed or manic episode

TX:
Medication and counseling
- Mood stabilizers
  - Examples:
    Lithium
    Valproic acid
    Carbamazepine
    Lamotrigine
- Antipsychotics
- Avoid stressful situations
- Regular sleep habits/exercise
- Good nutrition

Medical Reference Guide

PSYCHIATRY

Dementia

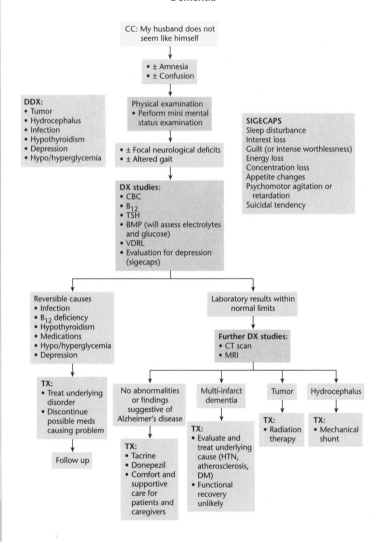

CC: My husband does not seem like himself

- ± Amnesia
- ± Confusion

DDX:
- Tumor
- Hydrocephalus
- Infection
- Hypothyroidism
- Depression
- Hypo/hyperglycemia

Physical examination
- Perform mini mental status examination

- ± Focal neurological deficits
- ± Altered gait

SIGECAPS
Sleep disturbance
Interest loss
Guilt (or intense worthlessness)
Energy loss
Concentration loss
Appetite changes
Psychomotor agitation or retardation
Suicidal tendency

DX studies:
- CBC
- B_{12}
- TSH
- BMP (will assess electrolytes and glucose)
- VDRL
- Evaluation for depression (sigecaps)

Reversible causes
- Infection
- B_{12} deficiency
- Hypothyroidism
- Medications
- Hypo/hyperglycemia
- Depression

Laboratory results within normal limits

Further DX studies:
- CT scan
- MRI

TX:
- Treat underlying disorder
- Discontinue possible meds causing problem

Follow up

No abnormalities or findings suggestive of Alzheimer's disease

TX:
- Tacrine
- Donepezil
- Comfort and supportive care for patients and caregivers

Multi-infarct dementia

TX:
- Evaluate and treat underlying cause (HTN, atherosclerosis, DM)
- Functional recovery unlikely

Tumor

TX:
- Radiation therapy

Hydrocephalus

TX:
- Mechanical shunt

PSYCHIATRY

Depression

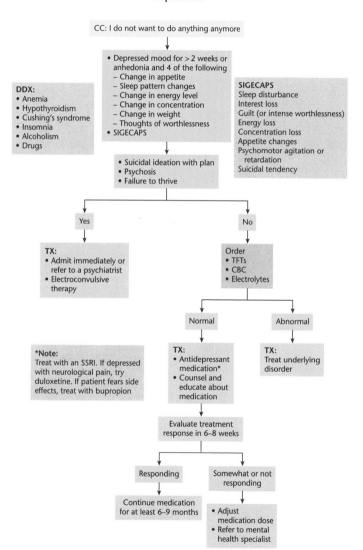

CC: I do not want to do anything anymore

- Depressed mood for > 2 weeks or anhedonia and 4 of the following
  - Change in appetite
  - Sleep pattern changes
  - Change in energy level
  - Change in concentration
  - Change in weight
  - Thoughts of worthlessness
- SIGECAPS

DDX:
- Anemia
- Hypothyroidism
- Cushing's syndrome
- Insomnia
- Alcoholism
- Drugs

SIGECAPS
Sleep disturbance
Interest loss
Guilt (or intense worthlessness)
Energy loss
Concentration loss
Appetite changes
Psychomotor agitation or retardation
Suicidal tendency

- Suicidal ideation with plan
- Psychosis
- Failure to thrive

Yes

No

TX:
- Admit immediately or refer to a psychiatrist
- Electroconvulsive therapy

Order
- TFTs
- CBC
- Electrolytes

Normal

Abnormal

*Note:
Treat with an SSRI. If depressed with neurological pain, try duloxetine. If patient fears side effects, treat with bupropion

TX:
- Antidepressant medication*
- Counsel and educate about medication

TX:
Treat underlying disorder

Evaluate treatment response in 6–8 weeks

Responding

Somewhat or not responding

Continue medication for at least 6–9 months

- Adjust medication dose
- Refer to mental health specialist

PSYCHIATRY

Psychosis

CC: My wife went crazy on me

Ensure safety of patient and others

- Altered mental state
- Delusional
- ± Hallucinations
- ± Combative

DX test:
- CBC
- BMP
- Ca^{2+}
- Mg^{2+}
- Phosphorus

- TSH
- Liver function
- B$_{12}$/folate
- UA
- Toxicology screen

Consider:
- *HIV test
- Hepatitis
- ANA
- Heavy metal screen
- Ceruloplasmin
- Porphobilinogens

>1 month but <6 month duration

Schizophreniform disorder

<1 month duration

Brief psychotic disorder

TX:
Antipsychotics
- ± Benzodiazepines
- Consider hospitalization

*Note:
Consider CT scan of the head in HIV patients to rule out toxoplasmosis and lymphoma

---

>6 month duration

Schizophrenia

See schizo algorithm for further evaluation page 111

>6 month duration with mood disorder

Schizoaffective disorder

TX:
- Mood stabilizers
  - Lithium
  - Carbamazepine
  - Valproate
- Antidepressants
- ECT
- Antipsychotics
- Consider hospitalization

Outpatient psychosocial treatments:
- Behavioral skills training
- Multifamily groups
- Partial hospital day treatment
- Vocational training/ sheltered workshops

- Fixed nonbizzare delusion for at least 1 month

TX:
Antipsychotics
- Hospitalization if necessary
- Psychotherapy
- Family psychoeducation

If an organic etiology is found

Treat underlying disorder

DDX:
- Psychosis
- Brief psychotic disorder
- Schizophreniform disorder
- Schizophrenia
- Schizoaffective disorder

PSYCHIATRY

Schizophrenia

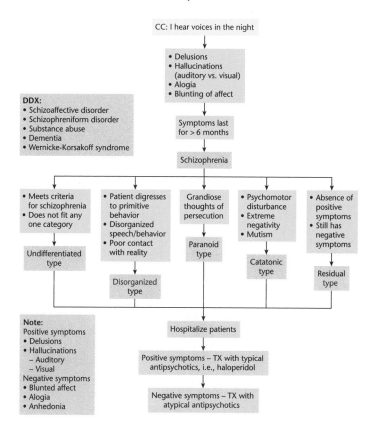

CC: I hear voices in the night

- Delusions
- Hallucinations (auditory vs. visual)
- Alogia
- Blunting of affect

DDX:
- Schizoaffective disorder
- Schizophreniform disorder
- Substance abuse
- Dementia
- Wernicke-Korsakoff syndrome

Symptoms last for > 6 months

Schizophrenia

- Meets criteria for schizophrenia
- Does not fit any one category

Undifferentiated type

- Patient digresses to primitive behavior
- Disorganized speech/behavior
- Poor contact with reality

Disorganized type

Grandiose thoughts of persecution

Paranoid type

- Psychomotor disturbance
- Extreme negativity
- Mutism

Catatonic type

- Absence of positive symptoms
- Still has negative symptoms

Residual type

Note:
Positive symptoms
- Delusions
- Hallucinations
  - Auditory
  - Visual
Negative symptoms
- Blunted affect
- Alogia
- Anhedonia

Hospitalize patients

Positive symptoms – TX with typical antipsychotics, i.e., haloperidol

Negative symptoms – TX with atypical antipsychotics

PSYCHIATRY

Substance Abuse

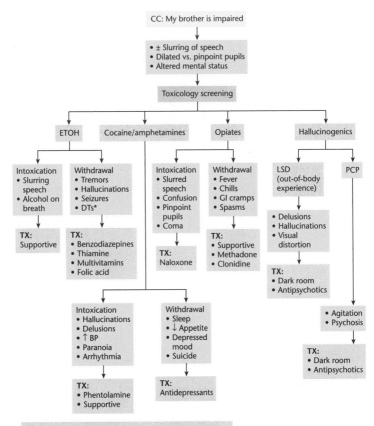

CC: My brother is impaired

- ± Slurring of speech
- Dilated vs. pinpoint pupils
- Altered mental status

Toxicology screening

ETOH

Intoxication
- Slurring speech
- Alcohol on breath

TX: Supportive

Withdrawal
- Tremors
- Hallucinations
- Seizures
- DTs*

TX:
- Benzodiazepines
- Thiamine
- Multivitamins
- Folic acid

Cocaine/amphetamines

Intoxication
- Hallucinations
- Delusions
- ↑ BP
- Paranoia
- Arrhythmia

TX:
- Phentolamine
- Supportive

Withdrawal
- Sleep
- ↓ Appetite
- Depressed mood
- Suicide

TX: Antidepressants

Opiates

Intoxication
- Slurred speech
- Confusion
- Pinpoint pupils
- Coma

TX: Naloxone

Withdrawal
- Fever
- Chills
- GI cramps
- Spasms

TX:
- Supportive
- Methadone
- Clonidine

Hallucinogenics

LSD (out-of-body experience)

- Delusions
- Hallucinations
- Visual distortion

TX:
- Dark room
- Antipsychotics

PCP

- Agitation
- Psychosis

TX:
- Dark room
- Antipsychotics

Note:
All patients with substance abuse/addiction should be given the option for counseling and drug rehabilitation

*DT = Delirium tremens

Frequently
Used Notes

Frequently Used Notes Categories

What is a SOAP Note?

In your clinical years as a medical student and physician, you will be responsible for taking detailed notes on the interactions you have with your patients. This is commonly done with a SOAP note, which stands for the following four parts:

SUBJECTIVE,

OBJECTIVE,

ASSESSMENT

PLAN

The general idea of a SOAP note is to **begin with the patient's chief complaint** and to continue to address this complaint throughout the above four parts. You should **write your SOAP note in your own words from your own observations.** Do not simply copy the previous note from an intern, resident, or student. It's better to write down what you heard from the patient and what results you collected from the physical examination.

Here are brief descriptions of each of the four parts:

S — Subjective: Simply put, this is the story the patient tells you in his/her own words. This should include the patient's chief complaint and other pertinent history, as well as any description of pain or other symptoms.

O — Objective: This is data that can be measured such as vital signs, physical examinations, laboratory data, X-ray results, EKGs, or any procedure performed to uncover the patient's condition.

A — Assessment: This is your interpretation of the patient's condition or level of progress. Basically, it is what you think is going on with the patient. It is not just a restatement of the patient's chief complaint. Your assessment will determine whether or not the patient's problem has been resolved or if further care will be required. You can also include differential diagnosis and working diagnosis, with the appropriate steps you may take to confirm or deny each of them.

P — Plan: The plan should include specific orders that will manage the patient's problems and complaints, as well as educational information and counseling for the patient and possibly the patient's family. It can also include an explanation of the treatments that are being carried out that day or treatments that may follow once a patient is discharged.

The rest of the chapter will provide guidelines for writing SOAP notes.

The Admit Note

This note is used to evaluate a patient at the beginning of an office visit or used as the first step in assessing a patient's reason for coming to the hospital. It encompasses a complete **history and physical examination**.

<u>**Date and time:**</u> It is best to write the complete date and time. (00/00/0000; 00:00 a.m./p.m.)

<u>**Source:**</u> of Hx and reliability

<u>**Chief complaint (CC):**</u> Reason the patient sought medical treatment

<u>**History of present illness (HPI):**</u> During your introduction to the patient, note the patient's age, race, gender, and the relevant information about the patient's medical problem in sequence of events. Include pertinent information from PMHx, risk factors, contributing factors, FH, SH, and ROS.

<u>**Allergies:**</u> Medication? Food? Reactions?

<u>**Medications:**</u> List the patient's medications, including the dosage and quantity taken (best confirmed by the patient's actual medication bottles). This also includes over-the-counter medications and any vitamins, herbs, and home remedies.

<u>**Past medical history (PMHx):**</u> Include medical illnesses (i.e., diabetes mellitus, hypertension), past hospitalizations, immunization history, psychiatric history.

<u>**Past surgical history:**</u> Surgeries in the past

<u>**SH:**</u>
    Patient's living situation
    Religion
    Educational background
    Occupation, place of employment
    Tobacco (what kind, how much, how often, and how long)
    Alcohol (what kind, how much, how often, and how long)
    Illicit drugs (what kind, how much, how often, and how long)

<u>**FH:**</u> Health status of immediate family members; the ages and possible causes of death of any deceased family members

Health-care proxy: A family member or close friend that the patient has appointed to make health-care decisions if he or she loses the ability to make decisions

Review of systems (ROS): An investigation into the functioning of all body systems:

General: changes in weight, changes in diet, weakness, fatigue, fever, chills, night sweats, changes in sleeping patterns

Dermatologic: itching, rashes, discoloration, moles, freckles, birthmarks, scars, lumps, bumps, bleeding, bruising, lesions, hair loss or gain, nail changes

Head: headache and location, dizziness, trauma, nausea, vomiting

Eyes: changes in vision in the past six months, use of contact lenses or glasses, double vision, floaters, sensitivity to light, blurring, itchiness, tearing, date of last eye examination

Ear: tinnitus, vertigo, hearing loss, use of hearing aids, discharge, past infections

Nose: epistaxis, discharge, stuffiness, sneezing, allergies

Mouth & Throat: dental disease, bleeding gums, dental caries, fillings, dentures, date of last dental examination, soreness, hoarseness

Neck: swollen neck, lumps, bumps, thyroid disease, stiffness

Respiratory: shortness of breath, wheezing, productive versus nonproductive cough, asthma, pneumonia, bronchitis, tuberculosis, emphysema, date of last chest X-ray

Cardiovascular: chest pain or pressure, angina, orthopnea, paroxysmal nocturnal dyspnea, dyspnea on exertion, murmurs, palpitations, hypertension, rheumatic fever, peripheral edema, date of last EKG

GI: appetite, dysphagia, abdominal pain, nausea, vomiting, GERD, diarrhea, constipation, melena, hematochezia, bowel movements (quantity and color change), jaundice, hepatitis, rectal bleeding, hemorrhoids

GU: dysuria, frequency, urgency, hesitancy, incontinence, hematuria, discharge, stones, urinary tract infection

Breast: lumps, trauma, tenderness, pain, nipple discharge, self breast examination/mammogram

Genital:

Male: penile discharge, pain, soreness, itching, testicular swelling, hernia, self testicular examination

Female: menarche, regularity, date of last menstrual period, number of pregnancies and children, abortions, birth control, menopause, hot flashes, itching, discharge, sores, vaginal bleeding

Male and Female: sexual interest, problems, sexually transmitted diseases, STD treatment, use of contraception

Endocrine: polyuria, polydipsia, heat or cold intolerance, thyroid problems, diabetes

Musculoskeletal: joint pain, swelling, arthritis, weakness, range of motion, broken bones, fractures, dislocation

Vascular: varicosities, leg edema, claudication, change in skin color, temperature, thickness or ulcerations

Neurological: loss of sensation, numbness, weakness, paralysis, tingling, tremors, blackouts, seizures, memory loss, problems with cognition, ataxia, loss of coordination, tremor, tics

Psychiatric: memory changes, depression, mood, anxiety, tension, suicidal ideation, problems maintaining relationships or jobs, hallucinations

Physical Examination: Include a complete examination of the entire body with focus on the area of complaint:

General: appearance, distress, behavior, cooperation, hygiene, brief assessment of mental status; A & O x 3 (person, place, time)

Vital Signs: current blood pressure, temperature, pulse, respirations, height, weight, oxygen saturation

Head: size, shape, trauma, TMJ, sensory and motor

Eyes: pupil size, shape, reactivity, visual fields and acuity, extraocular movement, scleral icterus, fundal papilledema

Ears: external ear, auditory acuity, tympanic membrane (dull, shiny, bulging, injected or intacted), tenderness

Nose: nasal discharge, sense of smell, symmetry, turbinate inflammation, frontal/maxillary sinus tenderness

Mouth &Throat: mucous membrane color and moisture, oral lesions, dentition, pharynx, tonsils, tongue, palate, uvula, exudates

Neck: lymphadenopathy, masses, carotid bruits, thyroid disease tracheal/spinal deviation, range of motion, shoulder shrug

Breasts: skin changes, symmetry, nipple discharge, masses, tenderness

Respiratory: clubbing, central cyanosis, equal expansion of the lungs, chest configuration, tactile fremitus, percussion, diaphragmatic excursion, auscultation (wheezing, crackles, egophony, rales, ronchi), tactile fremitus

Cardiovascular: S1, S2, gallops, rubs, murmurs, thrills, friction rubs, pulses, point of maximal impulse, heaves, heart span, carotid bruits, jugular venous distension, edema, varicose veins, carotid, radial, femoral, popliteal, posterior tibial, dorsalis pedis pulses

Abdomen: surgical scars, distention, bowel sounds, bruits, liver span, ascites, percussion, tenderness, masses, rebound, guarding (voluntary vs. nonvolutary), spleen size, costovertebral angle tenderness (CVA)

Urological: rashes, nodules, induration, ulcer, scars, discharge, hernias, varicoceles, scrotal masses, tenderness

Gynecological: inflammation, discharge, bleeding, ulcers, nodules, external genitalia, vaginal mucosa, cervix, uterine size and shape, adnexal masses, and ovaries

Rectal: sphincter tone, prostate consistency, masses, fissures, hemorrhoids, occult stool blood

Musculoskeletal: muscle atrophy, weakness, range of motion, instability, joint tenderness, crepitus, joint effusions, redness, swelling, spinal deviation, gait

Lymphatic: cervical, intraclavicular, acillary, trochlear, inguinal adenopathy

Neurological: cranial nerves, sensation, strength, reflexes, cerebellum, gait, weakness, seizures, numbness, tingling

Laboratory Results: Any laboratory and radiographic study results that have been performed upon admission as well as EKG results.

Assessment/Plan: The assessment can be an interpretation of the patient's condition or level of progress along with a differential diagnosis. The plan is based on the differential diagnosis and includes specific orders that will confirm or deny each of them (for example, ordering a chest X-ray on a patient with shortness of breath). It is also important to have educational information and counseling available for the patient if necessary. The plan should also include treatments and medications that may ease the patient's symptoms until many of the differential diagnoses are narrowed, along with an explanation of why they are being utilized.

Admission Orders

These orders are usually written directly after the admit note and are used to initially direct the patient's hospital stay. Use the following acronym to remember the orders' needed information.

(ADC VAAN DISML)

Date and time: It is best to write the complete date and time. (00/00/0000; 00:00 a.m./p.m.)

Admit/Transfer: Attending, Resident, Team, Floor, Room, Service

Diagnosis: In order of priority

Condition: good, fair, stable, guarded, critical, etc.

Vitals: Q4, Q shift, etc.

Allergies: List medications or types of food, NKDA, etc.

Activities: bed rest, ambulate 3 times a day, etc.

Nurse's Orders: I&O Foley to gravity, JP to bulb suction, NGT to intermittent suction, etc.

Diet: NPO, regular, diabetic, etc.

IVF: Lactated Ringer's or normal saline, maintenance ([D5 ½ NS + 20 KCL])

Special instructions: dressing changes, etc.

Meds: antibiotics, insulin, pain medication, O_2, anticoagulants, etc.

Labs: SMA-7, CBC with diff, +/− coags, etc.

Discharge Summary

This summary is given once it is agreed the patient no longer needs to be hospitalized.

Patient's Name:

Chart Number:

Date of Admission:

Date of Discharge:

Admitting Diagnosis:

Discharge Diagnosis:

Reason for Hospitalization:

Procedures: List surgical procedures, diagnostic tests, invasive procedures, etc.

Pertinent Physical Examination & Laboratory Data: Describe the course of the patient's illness/disease *before* being admitted to the hospital; include the pertinent physical examination and laboratory data.

Hospital Course: Describe the course of the patient's illness/disease while the patient was in the hospital. Include any evaluations, treatments, outcome of the treatments, and all medications given while in the hospital.

Discharge Condition: Describe any improvements or deteriorations in the patient's condition.

Disposition: Note where the patient will be discharged to (home, nursing home) and the person who will take care of the patient.

Discharge Medications: List medications with dosage, administration, refills.

Discharge Instructions & Follow-up Care: Note the date for follow-up care; diet, exercise, emergency phone numbers, etc.

Progress Note

This note is a continuation of the initial history and physical examination. It documents the patient's visit in the office as well as follows the patient throughout his or her stay in the hospital.

Medicine:

Date and time: It is best to write the complete date and time. (00/00/0000; 00:00 a.m./p.m.)

Subjective: Include the patient's age, gender, reasons for hospital visit, and date of admission. How is the patient feeling currently? Is he or she in any pain? If so, rate it on a scale of 1–10. Does the patient have any new complaints? Have prior symptoms been eliminated? You should also include a short focused review. (If your patient came in because of abdominal pain, ask questions pertaining to the abdomen.) Always include the cardiovascular and respiratory system. Ask about shortness of breath, chest pain, palpitations, change or blurring in vision, nausea, vomiting, diarrhea, and constipation.

Objective: These include the patient's vital signs as seen below. You can also include weight, height, and oxygen saturation, if necessary.

Temperature:

Pulse Rate:

Respiratory Rate:

Blood Pressure:

Laboratory results: Write the results for any labs such as CBC and SMA-7, as well as the results of any studies such as CT scans, X-rays, MRI's, and EKG's. If a study or blood work has been done and the results are not in, document that the results are pending. Laboratory results may be written in a skeleton format. Results can be written in skeleton format. If your patient is diabetic, then include the last three readings of his or her finger sticks.

Physical examination: For the SOAP note, the examination should always include the cardiovascular and respiratory system as well as a focused examination of the problem(s) being addressed. The admit note should encompass the complete physical examination.

Assessment/Plan: The assessment can be an interpretation of the patient's condition or level of progress along with a differential diagnosis. The plan is based on the differential diagnosis and includes specific orders that will confirm or deny each of them; for example, ordering a chest X-ray on a patient with shortness of breath. It is also important to have educational information and counseling available for the patient, if necessary. The plan should also include treatments and medications, which may ease the patient's symptoms until many of the differential diagnoses are narrowed, along with an explanation of why they are being utilized.

Consultation Note

This note is written by specialists in their respective fields. Whether it be GI, Cardio, Renal, Heme Onc, or ID, the format of the initial consult note is very similar to that of a history and physical note with a couple of modifications. At the beginning of the note, it is important to mention the reason for consultation and that the consulted physicians are thankful for the consult. Next, the note outlines the specialist's impressions and lists pertinent problems and symptoms found and being managed by the consultant. It also provides recommendations and a synopsis of the management plan. All of the specialists' follow-up notes are done in the form of a SOAP note. The following example is that of a **Gastrointestinal (GI) Consultation**.

Reason for consultation: Abnormal liver function tests and abdominal pain. Thank you for this consultation.

Date and time: It is best to write the complete date and time. (00/00/0000; 00:00 a.m./p.m.)

HPI: A 77 y/o Caucasian female presented to the ED with epigastric and RUQ pain since last evening. The patient denied any radiation and does not have any alleviating factors. She stated that food aggravated her pain and caused her to feel nauseated. She states that she vomited and denies any blood in her vomitus. Patient had a fever in the ED of 101.6° F and was given Tylenol 650 mg PO × 1.

The patient denied diarrhea, constipation, chest pain, shortness of breath, headache, or dizziness.

Past medical history:
1. H/O Liver abscess in 1998
2. COPD
3. Hypertension
4. Osteoporosis
5. Aortoiliac disease
6. H/O C-section

Allergies: NKDA

Medication List: Actonel, folic acid

Review of Symptoms: Please see HPI.

Social History: Patient smokes one pack per day; however she cut down and now smokes 5 cigarettes a day. Patient denies alcohol use and abuse. Patient also denies illicit drug use.

Family History: Non contributory

Vital Signs: Temperature 95.9°F, Pulse: 73 bpm, Respiratory Rate: 20, Blood Pressure: 100/61, O_2 Saturation 95% on 2L NC

Laboratory Results:

CXR: atelectasis/scarring

CT: Gallstones, diverticuli, renal vascular calcifications

*Na+:*134 K+: 3.8 Cl-:101 CO_2: 25 BUN: 17 Cr: 0.8 Glu: 97 WBC:12.5 Hb: 11.8 HCT: 35.0 PLT: 185 GGT:233 Amonia: 30.4 Lipase:35 Albumin: 4.0 Total Bilirubin: 2.6

Direct bilirubin: 1.9 Alk Phos: 237 AST: 240 ALT: 148 Hepatitis Panel: Negative

1st troponin: 0.01 2nd Troponin: 0.06

Physical Examination:

General: NAD

HEENT: NC/AT, PERRLA, EOMI, light reflex present in B/L tympanic membranes. No erythema in pharynx.

Neck: Supple

Cardiovascular system: Regular rate and rhythm no m/r/g

Lungs: B/L crackles in the bases

Abdomen: +BS, + tenderness in the epigastric and right-upper quadrant area with voluntary guarding, negative Murphy's sign

Extremities: Patient has palpable pedal pulses and is negative for edema.

Impression:

1. Abdominal pain (epigastric/RUQ)
2. COPD
3. Hypertension
4. Aortoiliac disease
5. H\O liver abscess

Recommendations: The 77 y/o Caucasian female with abdominal pain and increased LFTs likely has alcoholic hepatitis with biliary disease, a possibly ascending cholangitis because patient had fever, and has increased WBC count and RUQ pain. The primary medicine team completed RUQ U/S, and we will await the results. If the RUQ U/S is normal, we will consider doing an MRCP. If it is abnormal we will consider doing an ERCP and if cholecystic disease were present, it would be advisable to consult the surgical team for possible removal. Patient's troponins are elevated. Will order nitroglycerine as needed for chest pain and an EKG in the a.m.

Psychiatric Progress SOAP Note

This note differs from the previous notes because of its concentration on the patient's psychiatric and personal history. The assessment and plan also center on the axis diagnosis.

<u>**Subjective:**</u> Information that is specific for that patient and focuses on psychiatric history

<u>**Objective:**</u>

>*Vital signs:*
>
>*Mental Status Examination:* outline given below
>
>*Laboratory Results:* any blood work or radiographic studies that may have been completed

<u>**Assessment:**</u> This is usually the Axis I and II diagnosis given to the patient and/or how the patient is doing in relation to how he or she was behaving prior to this note.

<u>**Plan:**</u> What medications and why, also the symptoms they are covering and how they are going to be titrated for effectiveness. Also note any psychosocial treatment planning or group therapy. If warranted, discharge planning.

<u>**Axis Diagnosis:**</u>

AXIS I: List the psychiatric disorders.

AXIS II: List personality disorders and mental retardation.

AXIS III: List the physical and medical problems.

AXIS IV: List the social and environmental stressors and/or problems.

AXIS V: Global Assessment of Functioning (GAF) scale assesses the occupational, psychological, and social functioning of adults. The *Children's Global Assessment Scale* assesses those patients who are under the age of 18. Both of these scales have a score range of (0–100). The adult scale is shown below:

>*91–100:* Superior functioning in a number of different activities, life's problems never seem to get out of hand. No symptoms.
>
>*81–90:* Absent or minimal symptoms (test anxiety), generally good functioning in all areas, interested and involved in a large

number of activities, socially effective, generally satisfied with life, no more than everyday problems or concerns.

71–80: Symptoms are transient and expectable reactions to psychosocial stresses; there is slight impairment in social, occupational, or school functioning.

61–70: There are mild symptoms OR some difficulties in social, occupational, or school functioning, but generally the patient functions well and has had some meaningful interpersonal relationships.

51–60: Symptoms are moderate OR there are some moderate difficulties in social, occupational, or school functioning.

41–50: Symptoms are serious OR there are serious impairments in social, occupational, or school functioning.

31–40: There is some impairment in reality testing and/or communication or major impairment in a number of areas (work or school, family relations, judgment, thinking, mood).

21–30: Behavior is influenced by delusions or hallucinations OR severe impairment in communications or judgment OR inability to function in all areas.

11–20: There is some danger of hurting self or others OR the patient occasionally fails to maintain minimal personal hygiene OR gross impairment in communication.

1–10: There is persistent danger of severely hurting self or others OR persistent inability to maintain minimum personal hygiene OR serious suicidal act with clear expectation of death.

0: There is not enough information available to provide a GAF.

Mental Status Examination

The following is the basic outline for the mental status examination.

General Description:
1. Appearance
2. Overt behavior and psychomotor activity
3. Attitude

Mood and Affectivity:
1. Mood
2. Affect
3. Appropriateness affect

Speech Characteristics:
1. Relevant, incoherent, fluent

Perception:
1. Hallucinations or illusions

Thought Content and Mental Records:
1. Thought process
2. Thought content

Sensorium and Cognition:
1. Consciousness
2. Orientation and memory
3. Concentration and attention
4. Reading and writing
5. Visiospatial ability
6. Abstract thought
7. Information and intelligence

Impulsivity:
1. Behavioral history on impulse control

Judgment and Insight:
1. Ability of the patient to act appropriately

Reliability:
1. Physician's assessment of the patient's reliability in assessing his or her situation

The Mini-Mental Status Examination

This type of examination note is used for the quick assessment of mental status of a patient. It is used as a screening test in patients and can be added to any note. This test is scored out of a possible 30 points. A score of less than 25 suggests impairment and a score of less than 20 indicates a definite impairment.

Orientation:

- What is the year, season, month, day and date? (5 Points)
- Where are we (country, province, city, hospital, or floor)? (5 Points)

Registration:

- Name three items (pen, apple, table) and ask the patient to recall them immediately. A reminder to the patient should be given that he or she will be asked to recall the objects in a few moments. (3 Points)

Attention and Concentration:

- Serial 7's backwards from 100 (100, 93, 86, 79, 72) or spell 'WORLD' backwards

Recall:

- Ask patients to recall the three objects mentioned previously (pen, apple, and table). (3 Points)

Language:

- Point to and ask the patient to name a pencil and watch. (2 Points)
- Ask patient to repeat "no if's, and's, or but's." (2 Points)
- Ask patient to follow a 3-step command: "Take this piece of paper in your right hand, fold it in half, and return it to me." (3 Points)
- Ask patient to read and obey a command that you wrote on a piece of paper (close your eyes). (1 Point)
- Ask patient to write a sentence. (1 Point)
- Ask patient to copy a design (octagon, inverted triangle). (1 Point)

Surgery Notes

There are three types of surgical notes: the preoperative note, the operative note, and the postoperative note. The preoperative note is a quick assessment of the patient prior to surgical intervention; it often takes into consideration the consultation of other services that assess the patient's risk factors. The operative note is used to summarize the procedure that was performed and the result along with complications that may have occurred. The postoperative note is written as a SOAP note and focuses on the patient's progression to baseline functioning.

Preoperative Note

Date and time: It is best to write the complete date and time. (00/00/0000; 00:00 a.m./p.m.)

Preoperative Diagnosis:

Procedure Planned:

Type of Anesthesia Planned:

Laboratory Data: SMA7 or CHEM-7, which includes electrolytes, BUN, creatinine, and glucose; CBC; PT/PTT; UA; EKG; chest X-ray; type and screen or type and cross; liver function tests; ABG; CT/MRI scan; orders: NPO, preoperative antibiotics, and patient preparation for procedure; examples include any preps that may be needed for the skin or colon, etc.

Risk Factors: Cardiovascular, renal, pulmonary, hepatic, coagulopathic, nutritional risk factors

Consent: Patients must sign an informed consent, which is a documented explanation of the patient's risks and benefits of the procedure.

Allergies: Any drug allergies the patient may have

Major Medical Problems: A list of co-morbidities that the patient may have

Medications: List of medications that the patient is currently taking

Operative Note

This note is written immediately after the procedure. Use the following acronym to remember the needed information.

(PPP, AABCDEFF)

Date and time of the Procedure: It is best to write the complete date and time. (00/00/0000; 00:00 a.m./p.m.)

Preoperative Diagnosis:

Postoperative Diagnosis:

Procedure:

Anesthesia: General endotracheal anesthesia (GETA), laryngeal mask airway (LMA), local w/ sedation

Names of Surgeon and Assistants: Attending, residents, and medical students

Complications:

Condition: stable/unstable, intubated/extubated, transferred to the recovery room/ICU/regular floor

Drains: Types of drains used and their specific locations

Estimated Blood Loss (EBL): in cc's

Fluids and Blood Products Administered During Procedure: Type and amount

Specimens: Pathology specimens, cultures, blood samples

> (The order of the acronym below may vary.)
>
> **A**nesthesia (GETA, LMA, spinal, local w/ sedation)
> **A**ssessment/Plan (assessment and plan)
> **B**lade (Surgeon)
> **C**omplications
> **D**rains
> **E**BL
> **F**luids & U/O
> **F**indings (specimens)

Postoperative Note

Date and time: It is best to write the complete date and time. (00/00/0000; 00:00 a.m./p.m.)

Subjective: Mental status and subjective condition. Is the patient in pain? If so, how is it being controlled?

Vital Signs: Temperature, blood pressure, pulse, respirations, in some cases O_2 saturation

Physical Examination: Chest, lungs, abdomen, etc. Inspect the wound and any surgical dressings. Describe the condition of the drains, including the appearance and volume of the output.

Laboratory results: Any blood work, cytology, or radiographic studies

Impression: List pertinent problems and symptoms found.

Plan: This section describes the plan for the coming weeks based on what was found during the surgery, including post-anesthesia incentive spirometry and pain control.

Obstetrics and Gynecologic Notes

The notes for Obstetrics and Gynecology still follow the same format as the SOAP notes, except that the focus is mainly on the female reproductive organs, history of menarche, conception, and births.

Gynecologic Note

Date and time: It is best to write the complete date and time. (00/00/0000; 00:00 a.m./p.m.)

Patient: Name, age, gravidity/parity, chief complaint

HPI:

Past Medical History:

Past Surgical History:

Past Gynecologic History:

Menses: menarche, cycle duration and length, cycle heaviness, intermenstrual bleeding, dysmenorrhea, amenorrhea, and if relevant, menopause

Sexually transmitted infections:

Sexual history:

Birth control method:

Abnormal Pap smears and date of last Pap:

Postmenopausal women: ask about hot flashes, night sweats, vaginal dryness, and any use of hormone/estrogen replacement therapy.

Mammogram:

Past OB History: Date of delivery, gestational age, type of delivery, sex, birth weight, complications

Family History:

Allergies:

Medications:

Social History:

<u>**Physical Examination:**</u> Focused; including heart and lungs

<u>**Review of Systems:**</u>

<u>**Plan:**</u>

Obstetrics Notes

Admission to Labor and Delivery Note

<u>**Date and time:**</u> It is best to write the complete date and time. (00/00/0000; 00:00 a.m./p.m.)

<u>**HPI:**</u> An example is as follows: 28y/o G3P2 at 37W5D EGA presents with painful contractions since noon. Pt reports good fetal movement and denies rupture of membranes or vaginal bleeding.

<u>**LMP:**</u> Date reported by the patient

<u>**Estimated Date of Confinement (EDC):**</u>

<u>**Past GYN History:**</u>

Menarche/Regularity?

Length of menses in days?

Amount of menses? (Ask how many pads used?)

History of abnormal Pap smears?

History of sexually transmitted diseases?

<u>**Past OB History:**</u>

Date of delivery:

Gestational age:

Type of delivery:

Gender:

Birth weight:

Complications:

<u>**PMH:**</u>

<u>**Medications:**</u> PNV, FeSO$_4$

<u>**Allergies:**</u> No Known Drug Allergies (NKDA)

PSH: Tobacco/EtOH/Drugs

Prenatal Course:

1st visit:

Sono (date taken and EDC from sono):

BP range:

Weight gain:

Blood type and RH status:

Indirect Coombs Test:

PPD status and date taken:

Gonorrhea/Chlamydia and dates taken:

Hepatitis B status:

HIV status:

Group B Hemolytic Strep status and date taken:

Glucose Challenge Test (GCT)/Glucose Tolerance Test (GTT):

Physical Examination (focused):

Vital signs: Temp; BP; HR; RR

General: In moderate distress with uterine contractions

HEENT: PERRLA EOMI conjunctiva clear

Heart: Normal S1 and S2, no murmurs or gallops

Lungs: Clear to auscultation bilaterally

Abdomen: Gravid, fundus non-tender, fundal height 37cm

Leopold maneuvers: Fetus is vertex, estimated fetal weight 3300 gm

Sterile speculum examination: if indicated to rule out spontaneous rupture of membranes (SROM)

Sterile vaginal exam (SVE): dilatation/effacement/station)

Extremities: no cyanosis, clubbing or edema

Assessment: 28 y/o G3P2 at term, in labor fetal heart rate tracing (FHRT) reassuring intrauterine pregnancy (IUP) at 37 weeks' gestation; FHRT—Baseline 140's, accelerations present, no decelerations; contractions—q 4–5 min

Plan:

Admit to L&D
NPO except ice chips
IV—D5LR at 125 cc/hr
Continuous electronic fetal monitoring
CBC, T&S, RPR
Anticipate vaginal delivery
Educate the patient on risks, benefits, and alternatives

Delivery Note

Date and time: It is best to write the complete date and time. (00/00/0000; 00:00 a.m./p.m.)

Description: Patient was fully dilated and pushing. Prepped and draped in the usual sterile fashion. NSVD of a live female, 3000 gm and Apgars 9/9. Delivered LOA, no nuchal cord, light meconium. Nose and mouth bulb suctioned at perineum. The body was delivered without difficulty. The cord was clamped and cut, and the baby was handed to the nurse. Placenta delivered spontaneously, intact. Fundus firm with minimal bleeding. Placenta appears intact with 3 vessel cord. Cervix, vagina and perineum inspected and a small 2nd-degree perineal laceration was observed and repaired under local anesthesia with 2–0 and 3–0 chromic suture in the usual fashion. Homeostasis assured, and the patient was transferred to the recovery room in good condition. EBL was 350 cc.

Postpartum Note

Date and Time: It is best to write the complete date and time. (00/00/0000; 00:00 a.m./p.m.)

Subjective: Ask all your patients about the following.

Pain: Ask if they are feeling any cramps, perineal pain, and/or leg pain? Is the pain relieved with medication? Do they need more pain meds?

Lochia (vaginal bleeding): Are their any clots? How heavy is the bleeding? How many pads are they using? Vaginal discharge? Appetite? Sleep? Activity?

Breast feeding: Are they breast feeding or planning on breast feeding? How is it going? Is the baby latching on?

Contraception: What is their contraceptive plan? Include their relevant sexual history.

Objective: Take the patient's vital signs and give a focused physical examination including all of the following:

Heart: normal S1 and S2, no murmurs or gallops

Lungs: clear to auscultation bilaterally

Abdomen: bowel sounds, soft? nontender?

Breasts: Are they engorged? Are nipples cracking/is the skin intact? Mastitis?

C-section: Dressing on/off? Clean/dry/intact incision site?

Uterus: location of the uterine fundus—below umbilicus? Is it firm/tender?

Lochia: color, amount, how many pads? How old is the pad?

Perineum: visually inspect perineum—hematoma? edema? episiotomy? Are the sutures intact?

Extremities: Is there any edema? Homan's sign?

Postpartum labs: Hemoglobin or hematocrit?

Assessment/Plan:

General assessment—afebrile, doing well, tolerating diet

Perineal care—dermaplast, ice, betadine wash

Contraception plans (must discuss before the patient goes home)

Breast feeding? Any problems? Encourage.

Discharge and follow-up plan

Follow-up appointment (usually scheduled within 4–6 weeks postpartum)

Postoperative Cesarean Section Order/Note

Date and time: It is best to write the complete date and time. (00/00/0000; 00:00 a.m./p.m.)

Order: Admit to Recovery Room, then postpartum floor when stable

Diagnosis: Status post (s/p) primary low transverse cesarean section (LTCS) for failure to progress (FTP)

Condition: Stable

Diet: NPO

Allergies: None

Vitals: q 15 min till stable, and as per routine

Activity: Ambulate with assistance this p.m.

Nursing: Strict input and output (I&O), Foley to gravity, call MD for Temp >101°F, BP >150/90, <90/60, Pulse >100 beats/min, or Respirations <10 or >24 breaths per minute, encourage breast feeding, pad count, dressing checks, and incentive spirometry to bedside; encourage 10x/h.

IV: Lactated Ringer's (LR) or D5LR at 125 cc/hr, with 20 units of Pitocin × 1–2 liters

Labs: CBC in a.m.

Medications:

    Morphine sulfate 2mg IV q 2 hours prn pain
    Percocet 1–2 tabs PO q 4–6 hours prn pain, when tolerating
        PO well
    Vistaril 25 mg IM or PO q 6 hours prn nausea
    Ibuprofen 800 mg PO q 8 hours prn pain, when tolerating
        PO well
    Prophylactic antibiotics if indicated
    Thromboprohylaxis for high-risk patients
    RhoGAM, if Rh-negative

Cesarean Section Note

Date and Time: It is best to write the complete date and time. (00/00/0000; 00:00 a.m./p.m.)

Postoperative: POD#1

<u>**Subjective:**</u> Ask your patient about the following:

Pain:

Nausea/vomiting:

Passing flatus:

<u>**Objective:**</u> Take the patient's vital signs as well as input and output, and give a focused physical examination.

Heart: normal S1 and S2, no murmurs or gallops

Lungs: clear to auscultation bilaterally

Abdomen: bowel sounds, soft? nontender?

Breasts: are they engorged? Are the nipples cracking/is the skin intact? Mastitis?

C-section: dressing on/off? Clean/dry/intact incision site?

Uterus: location of the uterine fundus—below umbilicus? Is it firm/tender?

Lochia: color, amount, how many pads? How old is the pad?

Perineum: visually inspect perineum—Hematoma? Edema? Episiotomy? Are the sutures intact?

Extremities: Is there any edema? Homan's sign?

Postpartum labs: hemoglobin or hematocrit

<u>**Assessment/Plan:**</u> Postoperative day #1 (POD #1), status post (S/P), primary C/S. Patient is afebrile and is tolerating pain well with medication. Routine postoperative care includes the following:

- Discontinue Foley catheter
- Discontinue IV pain medications and change to per oral (PO) pain medications when tolerating PO
- Out of bed (OOB)
- Advance diet as tolerated; begin with clear liquids in the a.m. and regular in the p.m.
- Discontinue IV fluids when tolerating PO fluids
- Patient may shower
- Check CBC for any change in hemoglobin or hematocrit (which may indicate that a patient is anemic)

Pediatric Notes

Pediatric notes often encompass a few different components compared to the adult progress note and the admission note. Those components often include history of immunizations, the patient's birth history, current diet, whether or not the patient's baby was breast fed or formula fed, and developmental history.

The other difference in pediatrics is how the history is taken. It is usually gathered from the mother or guardian of the child. It is important to listen to these patients' parents or guardians as they often provide the key in the diagnosis and/or the next step in management of the patient.

Pediatric Admit Note

<u>CC:</u> the presenting complaint

<u>Source:</u> child/parent/guardian

<u>HPI:</u> This is a discussion of the presenting factors that led up to the problem, using the acronym OPQRSTUVW (see Mnemonics chapter). It should also include when the infant or child was last well. There should also be questions addressing any sick contacts. Important and too infrequently asked are questions concerning cultural or alternative remedies that were prepared or given to the child.

<u>Past Medical History:</u> This should include any past illnesses.

<u>Past Surgical History:</u> Past surgeries for the patient

<u>Immunizations:</u> This section should include the patient's past immunizations.

<u>Birth History:</u> This should indicate whether the birth was spontaneous or induced and provide reasons. Describe any labor problems and the duration or labor, which may hint at congenital or anatomical injuries. Note if the delivery was vaginal, forceps, or caesarian-section. Initial birth weight of the baby, APGAR score, and if the patient has had any jaundice, cyanosis, breathing problems, seizures, or other difficulties. Did the patient have to stay in the hospital for any reason

after birth, receive any treatments/medications, or did he/she go home with the mother?

Feeding History:

> *Neonate or younger infant:* Method of feeding the infant, whether breast or formula. If breast fed, the duration and any associated problems and if any supplementation was needed. If formula fed, the type, dilution, any formula changes. Also included should be feeding frequency and amount per feeding.

> *Older Infants:* This should include the age of introduction of solids and of what the patient's diet is composed. Any problems with difficulty feeding, regurgitation, colic or vomiting, and vitamins or fluoride supplements used.

Growth and Development: See the tables provided on pages 148–151. It is also important to also ask the question "what do you enjoy about your baby?" For adolescents, it is important to ask about school attendance and performance.

Family History: History of developmental delays, congenital abnormalities and/or any specific illnesses related to the patient's problem.

Social History: This should include home structure, parents' occupations, family dynamics, any pets, marital stability, support systems, financial problems (social assistance), recreational history of the child, any major or traumatic life events (deaths, accidents, divorce), and child's interests and activities. *Adolescents:* Should be asked about H.E.A.D.S.:

> *Home:* living arrangements, family issues, relationship with parents

> *Education:* school attendance and performance, relationship with teachers and classmates

> *Activities:* what the patient does after work or school

> *Drugs:* any types of alcohol or drugs that are used by the patient and peers

> *Sexuality:* any sexual activity, sexual orientation, history of sexually transmitted diseases; for females, age of menarche, regularity, dysmenorrheal, menorrhagia, vaginal discharge

Review of Systems:

General: This includes health, growth, activity level, weight, fatigue, and sleep.

Dermatologic: any rashes or discoloration of the skin

Head: headache or dizziness

Eyes: any changes in vision, does patient sit too close to television or books

Ear: any tinnitus, vertigo, hearing loss, otorrhea, otalgia

Nose: epistaxis, discharge or sinus disease

Mouth & Throat: dental disease, hoarseness or throat pain

Respiratory: shortness of breath, cough, productive versus nonproductive

Cardiovascular: Infant: fatigue or sweating during feeding, cyanosis; *Older Infant and Child:* syncope, murmurs, ability to keep up with peers; *Adolescents:* chest pain, orthopnea, paroxysmal nocturnal dyspnea, dyspnea on exertion

GI: dysphagia, abdominal pain, nausea, vomiting, diarrhea, constipation, melena, hematochezia

GU: dysuria, frequency of urination, hesitancy, hematuria, discharge

Gynecological: number of pregnancies and children, abortions, last menstrual period, age of menarche, menopause, vaginal bleeding, breast mass

Endocrine: polyuria, polydyspnea, heat or cold intolerance

Musculoskeletal: Joint pain, swelling, arthritis

Lymphatics: easy bruising, lymphadenopathy

Neuropsychiatric: weakness, seizures, paresthesia, memory changes, depression

Vital Signs: These include not only classic blood pressure, pulse, temperature, respirations, and O_2 saturation, but also height, weight, and head circumference. They can be plotted on a graph to compare growth trends. For infants, loss of 5 to 7% of birth weight in the first few days of life is considered normal.

<u>**Physical Examination:**</u> This should include a complete examination of the entire body with a thorough focus on the area of complaint.

General: Appearance, distress, behavior, cooperation, hygiene

Vital Signs: current blood pressure, temperature, pulse, respirations, height, weight, oxygen saturation

Head: size, shape, trauma, TMJ, sensory, and motor

Eyes: pupil size, shape, reactivity, visual fields and acuity, extraocular movement, scleral icterus, fundal papilledema

Ears: external ear, auditory acuity, tympanic membrane (dull, shiny, bulging, injected or intact), tenderness

Nose: nasal discharge, sense of smell, symmetry, turbinate inflammation, frontal/maxillary sinus tenderness

Mouth & Throat: mucus membrane color and moisture, oral lesions, dentition, pharynx, tonsils, tongue, palate, uvula, exudates

Neck: lymphadenopathy, masses, carotid or thyroid bruits, thyroid disease tracheal/spinal deviation, range of motion, shoulder shrug

Dermatologic: Inspect skin for acute skin changes, trauma, drainage, induration, erythema, and temperature changes.

Respiratory: clubbing, central cyanosis, equal expansion of the lungs, chest configuration, tactile fremitus, percussion, diaphragmatic excursion, auscultation (wheezing, crackles, egophony, rales, ronchi)

Cardiovascular: S1, S2, gallops, rubs, murmurs, thrills, friction rubs, pulses, point of maximal impulse, heaves, heart span, carotid bruits, jugular venous distension, edema, varicose veins, carotid, radial, femoral, popliteal, posterior tibial, dorsalis pedis pulses

Abdomen: surgical scars, distention, bowel sounds, bruits, liver span, ascites, percussion, tenderness, masses, rebound, guarding (voluntary versus involuntary), spleen size, costovertebral angle tenderness (CVA)

Musculoskeletal: muscle atrophy, weakness, range of motion, instability, joint tenderness, crepitus, joint effusions, redness, swelling, spinal deviation, gait

Lymphatic: cervical, intraclavicular, acillary, trochlear, inguinal adenopathy

Neurological: cranial nerves, sensation, strength, reflexes, cerebellum, gait, weakness, seizures, numbness, tingling

Assessment and Plan: The assessment can be an interpretation of the patient's condition or his or her level of progress along with a differential diagnosis. The plan is based on the differential diagnosis and includes specific orders that will confirm or deny each of them. It is also important to have educational information and counseling available for the parents/guardian if necessary. Any home remedies or alternative treatments should be addressed, especially if they interfere with medications. The plan should also include treatments and medications that may ease the patient's symptoms until many of the differential diagnoses are narrowed along with an explanation of why they are being utilized.

Medical Reference Guide

Table 1a: Pediatric Developmental Milestones (Birth–3 mo)

Age	Prone	Ventral	Supine	Visual
Newborn	Turns head, nose touches	Flexed around supporting hand	Flexed	Prefers face, doll's eyes, moves in cadence with sound
1 mo	Turns head, clears surface, chin up	Lifts head to plane of body	Relaxed in tonic neck, head lag	Watches person, follows moving object, may smile
2 mo	Lifts head and chest	Sustains head in plane of body	Tonic neck, head lag, follows 180°	Smiles on social contact, attends to voice, and coos
3 mo	Lifts head and chest, with arms extended	Lifts head above plane of body, with legs extended	Tonic neck, reaches at objects, may fail to grasp, less head lag, head bobs on sitting	Sustained social smile, listens to music, some vowel sounds, "aah"

Table 1b: Pediatric Developmental Milestones (4 mo–6 mo)

Age	Prone	Supine	Sit/Stand	Manipulate	Social
4 mo	Head to vertical, legs extended	Symmetrical posture, hands to midline, grasps objects, brings to mouth	No head lag, head steady, sits with truncal support; held erect, pushes with feet	Regards pellet	Laughs out loud, displeased if social contact broken
6 mo	Rolls over, pivots, may creep, crawl	Lifts head, rolls over, squirms	Sits with pelvic support, back rounded, leans forward on hands	Rakes at pellet, turns body to extend reach and grasp	Prefers mother, repetitive vowels

Table 1c: Pediatric Developmental Milestones (9 mo–12 mo)

Age	Sit/Stand	Locomotor	Manipulative	Cognitive	Social
9 mo	Sits alone, back straight	Creeps/crawls, "walks" with hands held	Pincer grasp assisted	Alert to sound of own name, object permanence	Peek-a-boo, bye-bye, repetitive consonant
12 mo	Cruises, may stand	Walks with one hand held	Unassisted pincer, releases on request, pellet into bottle	One or more words	Plays ball, adjusts posture to dressing

Table 1d: Pediatric Developmental Milestones (15 mo–24 mo)

Age	Locomotor	Large Object	Small Object	Crayon	Social
15 mo	Walks alone, crawls up stairs	3-cube tower	Dumps pellet if shown	Makes line, scribbles	Indicates by pointing, hugs parents
18 mo	Runs stiffly, sits on small chair, walks down stairs, one hand held	4-cube tower	Dumps pellet on request	Imitates stroke	Feeds self, 10 words, seeks help, "NO," body parts
24 mo	Runs well, up/down stairs (one step), opens doors, climbs on furniture, jumps in place (both feet off)	7-cube tower, 4-cube train	Threads shoelace	Imitates vertical stroke, circular, folds paper imitatively	Handles spoon well, helps undress, listens to stories, 30–50 words, 2–3 word sentences, "I," "you," parallel play

Table 1e: Pediatric Developmental Milestones (30 mo–60 mo)

Age	Motor	Manipulative	Crayon	Social
30 mo	Up stairs alternating feet, stand on one foot	9-cube tower, adds chimney to train	Imitates vertical/horizontal strokes, not cross, imitates circular stroke with closure	Refers to self as "I," knows name, helps put things away, pretends in play
36 mo	Down stairs, (alternating), broad jump (both feet), rides tricycle	10-cube tower, imitates 3-cube bridge	Imitates cross, copies circle, tries to draw person	Knows age and sex, counts 3 objects, understands taking turns
48 mo	Hops on one foot, throws ball overhand, climbs well	Copies 3-cube bridge	Copies cross, square, draws figure with head, 2–4 parts	Counts 4 objects, tells a story, group play, goes to toilet alone
60 mo	Skips		Copies triangle, draws figure, 8–10 parts	

Table 2: Reflexes

Reflex	Description	Appears	Disappears	CNS Origin
Moro	Extend head → extension, flexion of arms, legs	Birth	4–6 mo	Brain stem vestibular nuclei
Grasp	Finger in palm → hand, elbow, shoulder flexion	Birth	4–6 mo	Brain stem vestibular nuclei
Rooting	Cheek stimulus → turns mouth to that side	Birth	4–6 mo	Brain stem trigeminal system
Trunk incurvation	Withdrawal from stroking along ventral surface	Birth	6–9 mo	Spinal cord
Placing	Steps up when dorsum of foot stimulated	Birth	4–6 mo	Cerebral cortex
Tonic neck	Fencing posture when supine	Birth	4–6 mo	Brain stem vestibular nuclei
Parachute	Simulate fall → extends arms	6–8 mo	Never	Brain stem vestibular

Table 3: Normal Pediatric Heart Rate

Age	Normal Heart Rate	
	Average (BPM)	Mean (BPM)
Newborn–3 months	94–140	140
3 months–1 year	124–180	140
1–3 years	98–160	126
3–5 years	65–132	98
5–8 years	70–115	96
8–12 years	55–107	79

BPM = Beats per minute

Laboratory Values

Laboratory Skeletons

The following skeletons are commonly used to describe the laboratory
results within a patient note.

Hematologic

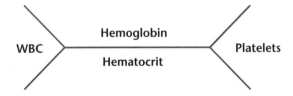

Chemistries

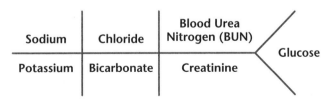

Arterial Blood Gases

PH / PaCO$_2$ / PaO$_2$ / HCO$_3$ / Oxygen Saturation / Base Excess

Hepatobiliary

Total Bilirubin	Alkaline Phosphatase	Aspartate Aminotransferase (AST)
Direct Bilirubin		Alanine Aminotransferase (ALT)

Coagulation Studies

Partial Thromboplastin Time (PTT) / Prothrombin Time (PT) / International Normalization Ratio (INR)

Medical Reference Guide

	REFERENCE RANGE	SI REFERENCE INTERVALS
BLOOD, PLASMA, SERUM		
Alanine aminotransferase (ALT, GPT at 30°C)	8–20 U/L	8–20 U/L
Alkaline phosphatase	41–133 units/L	0.7–2.2 µkat/L
Amylase, serum	25–125 U/L	25–125 U/L
Aspartate aminotransferase (AST, GOT at 30°C)	8–20 U/L	8–20 U/L
Bilirubin, serum (adult) Total // Direct	0.1–1.0 mg/dL // 0.0–0.3 mg/dL	2–17 µmol/L // 0–5 µmol/L
Calcium, serum (Total)	8.4–10.2 mg/dL	2.1–2.8 mmol/L
Cholesterol, serum	140–250 mg/dL	3.6–6.5 mmol/L
Cortisol, serum	0800 h: 5–23 µg/dL // 1600 h: 3–15 µg/dL 2000 h: 50% of 0800 h	138–635 nmol/L // 82–413 nmol/L Fraction of 0800 h: ≤ 0.50
Creatine kinase, serum (at 30°C) ambulatory	Male: 25–90 U/L Female: 10–70 U/L	25–90 U/L 10–70 U/L
Creatinine, serum	0.6–1.2 mg/dL	53–106 µmol/L
Electrolytes, serum		
Sodium	135–147 mEq/L	135–147 mmol/L
Chloride	95–105 mEq/L	95–105 mmol/L
Potassium	3.5–5.0 mEq/L	3.5–5.0 mmol/L
Bicarbonate	22–28 mEq/L	22–28 mmol/L
Estriol (E3) total, serum (in pregnancy)		
24–28 weeks // 32–36 weeks	30–170 ng/mL // 60–280 ng/mL	104–590 // 208–970 mmol/L
28–32 weeks // 36–40 weeks	40–220 ng/mL // 80–350 ng/mL	140–760 // 280–1210 mmol/L
Ferritin, serum	Male: 15–200 ng/mL Female: 12–150 ng/mL	15–200 µg/L 12–150 µg/L
Follicle–stimulating hormone, serum/plasma	Male: 4–25 mIU/mL Female: premenopause 4–30 mIU/mL	4–25 U/L 4–30 U/L
	midcycle peak 10–90 mIU/mL	10–90 U/L
	postmenopause 40–250 mIU/mL	40–250 U/L

Laboratory Values

	REFERENCE RANGE	SI REFERENCE INTERVALS
BLOOD, PLASMA, SERUM *(continued)*		
Gases, arterial blood (room air)		
pO₂	75–105 mm Hg	10.0–14.0 kPa
pCO₂	33–44 mm Hg	4.4–5.9 kPa
pH	7.35–7.45	[H⁺] 36–44 nmol/L
Glucose, serum	Fasting: 70–110 mg/dL	3.8–6.1 mmol/L
	2-h postprandial: < 120 mg/dL	< 6.6 mmol/L
Growth hormone — arginine stimulation	Fasting: < 5 ng/mL	< 5 µg/L
	provocative stimuli: < 7 ng/mL	<7 µg/L
Immunoglobulins, serum		
IgA	76–390 mg/dL	0.76–3.90 g/L
IgE	0–380 IU/mL	0–380 kIU/mL
IgG	650–1500 mg/dL	6.5–15 g/L
IgM	40–345 mg/dL	0.4–3.45 g/L
Iron	50–170 µg/dL	9–30 µmol/L
Lactate dehydrogenase (L → P, 30°C)	45–90 U/L	45–90 U/L
Luteinizing hormone, serum/plasma	Male: 6–23 mIU/mL	6–23 U/L
	Female: follicular phase 5–30 mIU/mL	5–30 U/L
	midcycle 75–150 mIU/mL	75–150 U/L
	postmenopause 30–200 mIU/mL	30–200 U/L
Osmolality, serum	275–295 mOsmol/kg	275–295 mOsmol/kg
Parathyroid hormone, serum, N-terminal	230–630 pg/mL	230–630 ng/L
Phosphatase (alkaline), serum (p-NPP at 30°C)	20–70 U/L	20–70 U/L
Phosphorus (inorganic), serum	3.0–4.5 mg/dL	1.0–1.5 mmol/L
Prolactin, serum (hPRL)	< 20 ng/mL	< 20 µg/L

Medical Reference Guide

	REFERENCE RANGE	SI REFERENCE INTERVALS
BLOOD, PLASMA, SERUM *(continued)*		
Proteins, serum		
Total (recumbent)	6.0–7.8 g/dL	60–78 g/L
Albumin	3.5–5.5 g/gL	35–55 g/L
Globulins	2.3–3.5 g/dL	23–35 g/L
Thyroid-stimulating hormone, serum or plasma	0.5–5.0 µU/mL	0.5–5.0 mU/L
Thyroidal iodine (^{123}I) uptake	8–30% of administered dose/24 h	0.08–0.30/24 h
Thyroxine (T_4), serum	5–12 µg/dL	64–155 nmol/L
Triglycerides, serum	35–160 mg/dL	0.4–1.81 mmol/L
Triiodothyronine (T_3), serum (RIA)	115–190 ng/dL	1.8–2.9 nmol/L
Triiodothyronine (T_3), resin uptake	25–35%	0.25–0.35
Urea nitrogen, serum (BUN)	7–18 mg/dL	1.2–3.0 mmol urea/L
Uric acid, serum	3.0–8.2 mg/dL	0.18–0.48 mmol/L
CEREBROSPINAL FLUID		
Cell count	0–5 cells/mm^3	0–5 x 10^6/L
Chloride	118–132 mmol/L	118–132 mmol/L
Gamma globulin	3–12% total proteins	0.03–0.12
Glucose	40–70 mg/dL	2.2–3.9 mmol/L
Pressure	70–180 mm H_2O	70–180 mm H_2O
Proteins, total	< 40 mg/dL	< 0.40 g/L
HEMATOLOGIC		
Bleeding time (template)	2–7 minutes	2–7 minutes
Erythrocyte count	Male: 4.3–5.9 million/mm^3 Female: 3.5–5.5 million/mm^3	4.3–5.9 × 10^{12}/L 3.5–5.5 × 10^{12}/L
Hematocrit	Male: 41–53% Female: 36–46%	0.41–0.53 0.36–0.46

	REFERENCE RANGE	SI REFERENCE INTERVALS
HEMATOLOGIC *(continued)*		
Hemoglobin, blood	Male: 13.5–17.5 g/dL	2.09–2.71 mmol/L
	Female: 12.0–16.0 g/dL	1.86–2.48 mmol/L
Hemoglobin, plasma	1–4 mg/dL	0.16–0.62 mmol/L
Leukocyte count and differential		
Leukocyte count	4500–11,000/mm^3	4.5–11.0 x 10^9/L
Segmented neutrophils	54–62%	0.54–0.62
Band forms	3–5%	0.03–0.05
Eosinophils	1–3%	0.01–0.03
Basophils	0–0.75%	0–0.0075
Lymphocytes	25–33%	0.25–0.33
Monocytes	3–7%	0.03–0.07
Mean corpuscular hemoglobin	25.4–34.6 pg/cell	0.39–0.54 fmol/cell
Mean corpuscular hemoglobin concentration	31–36% Hb/cell	4.81–5.58 mmol Hb/L
Mean corpuscular volume	80–100 µm^3	80–100 fl
Partial thromboplastin time (nonactivated)	60–85 seconds	60–85 seconds
Platelet count	150,000–400,000/mm^3	150–400 x 10^9/L
Prothrombin time	11–15 seconds	11–15 seconds
Reticulocyte count	0.5–1.5% of red cells	0.005–0.015
Sedimentation rate, erythrocyte (Westergren)	Male: 0–15 mm/h	0–15 mm/h
	Female: 0–20 mm/h	0–20 mm/h
Thrombin time	< 2 seconds deviation from control	< 2 seconds deviation from control
Volume		
Plasma	Male: 25–43 mL/kg	0.025–0.043 L/kg
	Female: 28–45 mL/kg	0.028–0.045 L/kg
Red cell	Male: 20–36 mL/kg	0.020–0.036 L/kg
	Female: 19–31 mL/kg	0.019–0.031 L/kg

Medical Reference Guide

	REFERENCE RANGE	SI REFERENCE INTERVALS
SWEAT		
Chloride	0–35 mmol/L	0–35 mmol/L
URINE		
Calcium	100–300 mg/24 h	2.5–7.5 mmol/24 h
Chloride	Varies with intake	Varies with intake
Creatinine clearance	Male: 97–137 mL/min Female: 88–128 mL/min	
Estriol, total (in pregnancy)		
30 weeks	6–18 mg/24 h	21–62 µmol/24 h
35 weeks	9–28 mg/24 h	31–97 µmol/24 h
40 weeks	13–42 mg/24 h	45–146 µmol/24 h
17-Hydroxycorticosteriods	Male: 3.0–10.0 mg/24 h Female: 2.0–8.0 mg/24 h	8.2–27.6 µmol/24 h 5.5–22.0 µmol/24 h
17-Ketosteriods, total	Male: 8–20 mg/24 h Female: 6–15 mg/24 h	28–70 µmol/24 h 21–52 µmol/24 h
Osmolality	50–1400 mOsmol/kg	
Oxalate	8–40 µg/mL	90–445 µmol/L
Potassium	Varies with diet	Varies with diet
Proteins, total	< 150 mg/24 h	< 0.15 g/24 h
Sodium	Varies with diet	Varies with diet
Uric acid	Varies with diet	Varies with diet

Medical Mnemonics

Medical Mnemonics Categories

Cardiology

CHF: causes of exacerbation
FAILURE

Forgot medication
Arrhythmia/**A**nemia
Ischemia/**I**nfarction/**I**nfection
Lifestyle: taken too much salt
Upregulation of cardiac output: pregnancy, hyperthyroidism
Renal failure
Embolism: pulmonary

MI: therapeutic treatment
MONAH

Morphine
Oxygen
Nitrogen
Aspirin
Heparin

Beck's triad (cardiac tamponade)
3 D's

Distant heart sounds
Distended jugular veins
Decreased arterial pressure

Jugular venous pressure (JVP) elevation: causes
HOLT

Heart failure
Obstruction of vena cava
Lymphatic enlargement—supraclavicular
Intra-**T**horacic pressure increase

Murmurs: right versus left loudness
RILE

Right-sided heart murmurs are louder on **I**nspiration.
Left-sided heart murmurs are loudest on **E**xpiration.

Murmurs: innocent murmur features
8 S's
Soft
Systolic
Short
Sounds (S1 and S2) normal
Symptomless
Special tests normal (X-ray, EKG)
Standing/**S**itting (vary with position)
Sternal depression

Heart murmur: attributes
Listen for the IL PQRST
Intensity
Location
Pitch
Quality
Radiation
Shape
Timing

Murmurs: systolic versus diastolic
PASS
Pulmonic and **A**ortic **S**tenosis = **S**ystolic
PAID
Pulmonic and **A**ortic **I**nsufficiency = **D**iastolic

Murmurs: locations and descriptions
MRS. A$$
MRS.: **M**itral **R**egurgitation—**S**ystolic
A$$: **A**ortic **S**tenosis—**S**ystolic

The other two murmurs, mitral stenosis and aortic regurgitation, are diastolic.

Aortic stenosis: characteristics
SAD
Syncope
Angina
Dyspnea

Aortic regurgitation: causes
CREAMS
Congenital
Rheumatic fever/**R**heumatoid arthritis
Endocarditis
Aortic dissection/**A**ortic root dilatation/**A**nkylosing spondylitis
Marfan's
Syphilis

MI: signs and symptoms
PULSE
Persistent chest pains
Upset stomach
Lightheadedness
Shortness of breath
Excessive sweating

EKG: 12-lead EKG quick interpretation of V1–V6
SSAALL
ST-wave changes in the following leads matched with
their classic location of MI:

V1 **S**eptal
V2 **S**eptal
V3 **A**nterior
V4 **A**nterior
V5 **L**ateral
V6 **L**ateral

EKG: T-wave inversion: causes
INVERT
Ischemia
Normality (especially in young, black patients)
Ventricular hypertrophy
Ectopic foci (calcified plaques)
RBBB, LBBB
Treatments (example: digoxin)

ST-elevation causes in ECG
ELEVATION
Electrolytes
LBBB
Early repolarization
Ventricular hypertrophy
Aneurysm
Treatment (pericardiocentesis)
Injury (AMI, contusion)
Osborne waves (hypothermia)
Non-occlusive vasospasm

Depressed ST-segment: causes
DEPRESSED ST
Drooping valve (MVP)
Enlargement of LV with strain
Potassium loss (hypokalemia)
Reciprocal ST-depression (in I/W AMI)
Embolism in lungs (pulmonary embolism)
Subendocardial ischemia
Subendocardial infarct
Encephalon hemorrhage (intracranial hemorrhage)
Dilated cardiomyopathy
Shock
Toxicity of digitalis, quinidine

Supraventricular tachycardia: treatment
ABCDE
Adenosine
Beta-blocker
Calcium channel antagonist
Digoxin
Excitation (vagal stimulation)

Ventricular tachycardia: treatment
LAMB
Lidocaine
Amiodarone
Mexiltene/**M**agnesium
Beta-blocker

Sinus tachycardia: causes
TACH FEVER

Tamponade/**T**hyrotoxicosis
Anemia
CHF
Hypotension
Fever
Excruciating pain
Volume depletion
Exercise
Rx (Theo, Dopa, Epi, etc.)

Sinus bradycardia: etiology
SINUS BRADICARDIA (sinus bradycardia)

Sleep
Infections (myocarditis)
Neap thyroid (hypothyroid)
Unconsciousness (vasovagal syncope)
Subnormal temperatures (hypothermia)
Biliary obstruction
Raised CO_2 (hypercapnia)
Acidosis
Deficient blood sugar (hypoglycemia)
Imbalance of electrolytes
Cushing's reflex (raised ICP)
Aging
Rx (drugs, such as high-dose atropine)
Deep anaesthesia
Ischemic heart disease
Athletes

Atrial fibrillation: causes
PIRATES

Pulmonary: PE, COPD
Iatrogenic
Rheumatic heart: mitral regurgitation
Atherosclerotic: MI, CAD
Thyroid: hyperthyroid
Endocarditis
Sick sinus syndrome

Atrial fibrillation: management

ABCD

Anticoagulate
Beta-block to control rate
Cardiovert
Digoxin

Anti-arrhythmics for AV nodes

Do Block AV

Digoxin
B-blockers
Adenosine
Verapamil

Pulseless electrical activity: causes

PATCH MED

Pulmonary embolus
Acidosis
Tension pneumothorax
Cardiac tamponade
Hypokalemia/**H**yperkalemia/**H**ypoxia/**H**ypothermia/**H**ypovolemia
Myocardial infarction
Electrolyte derangements
Drugs

Heart failure: signs

TAPED TORCH

Tachycardia
Ascites
Pulsus alternans
Elevated jugular venous pressure
Displaced apex beat
Third heart sound
Oedema
Right ventricular heave
Crepitations or wheeze
Hepatomegaly (tender)

Coronary artery bypass graft: indications
DUST

Depressed ventricular function
Unstable angina
Stenosis of the left main stem
Triple vessel disease

Peripheral vascular insufficiency: inspection criteria
SICVD

Symmetry of leg musculature
Integrity of skin
Color of toenails
Varicose veins
Distribution of hair

Rheumatic fever: revised Jones' criteria
JONES crITERIA

Major criteria:
Joint (arthritis)
Obvious (cardiac)
Nodule (rheumatic)
Erythema marginatum
Sydenham chorea
Minor criteria:
Inflammatory cells (leukocytosis)
Temperature (fever)
ESR/CRP elevated
Raised PR interval
Itself (previous Hx of rheumatic fever)
Arthralgia

Pericarditis: causes
PR DIP, ST UP

Post-pericardiectomy
Rheumatic fever
Drugs (examples: isoniazid, hydralazine, procainamide)
Infection (examples: TB, coxsackie, strep)
PE
SLE/**S**cleroderma
Tumors/**Th**yroid disease
Uremia
Post MI (includes Dressler's)

Aortic dissection: risk factors
ABC
Atherosclerosis/**A**geing/**A**ortic aneurysm
Blood pressure high/**B**aby (pregnancy)
Connective tissue disorders (examples: Marfan's, Ehlers-Danlos)/
   Cystic medial necrosis

Heart failure: causes
HEART FAILED
Hypertension
Endocrine
Anemia
Rheumatic heart disease
Toxins
Failure to take medications
Arrhythmia
Infection
Lung (PE, pneumonia)
Electrolytes
Diet

Dyspnea: causes
SHE PANTS
Stress, anxiety
Heart disease
Emboli
Pulmonary disease
Anemia
Neuromuscular disease
Trachea obstruction
Sleep disorder

Cyanosis: differential diagnosis
COLD PALMS

Peripheral cyanosis:
Cold
Obstruction
LVF and shock
Decreased cardiac output

Central cyanosis:
Polycythemia
Altitude
Lung disease
Met-, sulfhemoglobinemia
Shunt

Exercise contraindications
RAMP

Recent MI
Aortic stenosis
MI in the last 7 days
Pulmonary hypertension

Endocrine

Diabetic ketoacidosis: precipitating factors
5 I's
Infection
Ischemia (cardiac, mesenteric)
Infarction
Ignorance (poor control, noncompliance)
Intoxication (alcohol)

Hypoglycemia: causes
Let's EXPLAIN hypoglycemia.
EXogenous drugs (insulin, oral hypoglycemics, alcohol, pentamidine, quinine, quinolones)
Pituitary insufficiency (no GH or cortisol)
Liver failure (no glycogen stores)
Adrenal failure (no cortisol)
Insulinomas/**I**mmune hypoglycemia
Non-pancreatic neoplasms (retroperitoneal sarcoma)

Hypernatremia: causes
6 D's
Diuretics
Dehydration
Diabetes insipidus
Docs (iatrogenic)
Diarrhea
Disease: (examples: kidney, sickle cell)

Hypercalcemia: differential
VITAMIN TRAPS

Vitamin A and D intoxication
Immobilization
Thyrotoxicosis
Addison's disease/**A**cidosis
Milk-alkali syndrome
Inflammatory disorders
Neoplastic disease
Thiazides, other drugs
Rhabdomyolysis
AIDS
Paget's disease/**P**arenteral nutrition/**P**arathyroid disease
Sarcoidosis

SIADH: major signs and symptoms
SIADH

Spasms
Is pitting edema
Anorexia
Disorientation (and other psychoses)
Hyponatremia

SIADH: causes
SIADH

Surgery
Intracranial: infection, head injury, CVA
Alveolar: CA, pus
Drugs: opiates, antiepileptics, cytotoxics, antipsychotics
Hormonal: hypothyroid, low corticosteroid level

Acromegaly: symptoms
ABCDEF

Arthralgia/**A**rthritis
Blood pressure, raised
Carpal tunnel syndrome
Diabetes
Enlarged organs
Field defect

Short stature: causes
RETARD HEIGHT
Rickets
Endocrine (cretinism, hypopituitarism, Cushing's)
Turner syndrome
Achondroplasia
Respiratory (suppurative lung disease)
Down syndrome
Hereditary
Environmental (post-irradiation, post-infectious)
IUGR
GI (malabsorption)
Heart (congenital heart disease)
Tilted backbone (scoliosis)

Gynecomastia: common causes
GYNECOMASTIA
Genetic disorder (Klinefelter)
Young boy (pubertal)
Neonate
Estrogen
Cirrhosis/**C**imetidine/**CA**$^{++}$ channel blockers
Old age
Marijuana
Alcoholism
Spironolactone
Tumors (testicular and adrenal)
Isoniazid/**I**nhibition of testosterone
Antineoplastics (alkylating agents)/**A**ntifungal (ketoconazole)

Carcinoid syndrome: features
FACADE
Flushing
Asthma
Cor pulmonale
Ascites
Diarrhea
Endocardial fibrosis

Malaise and lethargy: causes
FATIGUED

Fat/**F**ood (poor diet)
Anemia
Tumor
Infection (HIV, endocarditis)
General joint or liver disease
Uremia
Endocrine (Addison's, myxedema)
Diabetes/**D**epression/**D**rugs

Gastrointestinal

Dry mouth: differential
DRI
Drugs/**D**ehydration
Renal failure/**R**adiotherapy
Immunological (Sjögren's)/**I**ntense emotions

Dysphagia: differential
DISPHAGIA
Disease of mouth and tonsils/**D**iffuse esophageal spasm
   Diabetes mellitus
Intrinsic lesion
Scleroderma
Pharyngeal disorders/**P**alsy-bulbar-MND
Heart: left atrium enlargement
Achalasia
Goiter/myasthenia **G**ravis/mediastinal **G**lands
Infections
American trypanosomiasis (Chagas' disease)

Dysphagia: causes
MOON
Mouth lesions
Obstruction
Oesophageal stricture
Neurological (examples: stroke, Guillain-Barré, achalasia)

Vomiting extra GI: differential
VOMITING
Vestibular disturbance/**V**agal (reflex pain)
Opiates
Migraine/**M**etabolic (DKA, gastroparesis, hypercalcemia)
Infections
Toxicity (cytotoxic, digitalis toxicity)
Increased ICP, **I**ngested alcohol
Neurogenic, psychogenic
Gestation

Hemoptysis: causes
HEMOPTYSIS

Hemorrhagic diathesis
Edema (LVF due to mitral stenosis)
Malignancy
Others (example: vasculitis)
Pulmonary vascular abnormalities
Trauma
Your treatment (anticoagulants)
SLE
Infarction in lungs
Septic

Hemoptysis: causes
CAVITATES

CHF
Airway disease, bronchiectasis
Vasculitis/**V**ascular malformations
Infection (example: TB)
Trauma
Anticoagulation
Tumor
Embolism
Stomach

Vomiting: non-GI differential
ABCDEFGHI

Acute renal failure
Brain (increased ICP)
Cardiac (inferior MI)
DKA
Ears (labyrinthitis)
Foreign substances (examples: Tylenol, Theophylline)
Glaucoma
Hyperemesis gravidarum
Infection (pyelonephritis, meningitis)

Abdomen: assessment

To assess abdomen, palpate all 4 quadrants for DR. GERM.

Distension: liver problems, bowel obstruction
Rigidity (board like): bleeding
Guarding: muscular tension when touched
Evisceration/**E**cchymosis
Rebound tenderness: infection
Masses

Abdominal swelling: causes

9 F's

Fat
Feces
Fluid
Flatus
Fetus
Full-sized tumors
Full bladder
Fibroids
False pregnancy

Abdominal pain: medical causes

ABDOMENAL PANE (abdominal pain)

Acute rheumatic fever
Blood (purpura, a/c hemolytic crisis)
DKA
c**O**llagen vascular disease
Migraine (abdominal migraine)
Epilepsy (abdominal epilepsy)
Nephron (uremia)
Abdominal angina
Lead
Porphyria
Arsenic
NSAIDs
Enteric fever

Left-quadrant abdominal pain: medical causes
SUPER CLOT

Sigmoid diverticulitis
Uteric colic
PID
Ectopic pregnancy
Rectus sheath hematoma
Colorectal carcinoma
Left-sided, lower-lobe pneumonia
Ovarian cyst (rupture, torture)
Threatened abortion/**T**esticular torsion

IBD: extraintestinal manifestations
A PIE SAC

Aphthous ulcers
Pyoderma gangrenosum
Iritis
Erythema nodosum
Sclerosing cholangitis
Arthritis
Clubbing of fingertips

Bilirubin: common causes for increased levels
HOT Liver

Hemolysis
Obstruction
Tumor
Liver disease

Charcot's triad (gallstones): features
3 C's

Color change (jaundice)
Colic (biliary) pain (RUQ pain)
Chills and fever

Cholangitis: features
CHOLANGITIS
Charcot's triad/**C**onjugated bilirubin increase
Hepatic abscesses/**H**epatic (intra/extra) bile ducts/**H**LA B8, DR3
Obstruction
Leukocytosis
Alkaline phosphatase increase
Neoplasms
Gallstones
Inflammatory bowel disease (ulcerative colitis)
Transaminase increase
Infection
Sclerosing

Pancreatitis (acute): causes
I GET SMASHED.
Idiopathic
Gallstones
Ethanol
Trauma
Steroids
Mumps
Autoimmune (PAN)
Scorpion stings
Hyperlipidemia/**H**ypercalcemia
ERCP
Drugs (including azathioprine and diuretics)

Pancreatitis: Ranson criteria for pancreatitis: at admission
GA LAW
Glucose >200
AST > 250
LDH > 350
Age > 55 yo
WBC > 16,000

Liver failure: decompensating chronic liver failure: differential
HEPATICUS

Hemorrhage
Electrolyte disturbance
Protein load
Alcohol binge
Trauma
Infection
Constipation
Uremia
Sedatives/**S**hunt/**S**urgery

Hepatic encephalopathy: precipitating factors
HEPATICS

Hemorrhage in GIT/**H**yperkalemia
Excess protein in diet
Paracentesis
Acidosis/**A**nemia
Trauma
Infection
Colon surgery
Sedatives

Chronic liver failure: signs found on the upper limbs
CLAPS

Clubbing
Leukonychia
Asterixis
Palmar erythema
Scratch marks

Crohn's disease morphology: symptoms

CHRISTMAS

Cobblestones
High temperature
Reduced lumen
Intestinal fistulae
Skip lesions
Transmural (all layers, may ulcerate)
Malabsorption
Abdominal pain
Submucosal fibrosis

Ulcerative colitis: definition of a severe attack

A STATE

Anemia less than 10g/dL
Stool frequency greater than 6 stools with blood/day
Temperature greater than 37.5°C
Albumin less than 30g/L
Tachycardia greater than 90 bpm
ESR greater than 30 mm/hr

Ulcerative colitis: complications

PAST Colitis

Pyoderma gangrenosum
Ankylosing spondylitis
Sclerosing pericholangitis
Toxic megacolon
Colon carcinoma

Digestive disorders: pH level

With vomiting, both the pH and food come up.
With diarrhea, both the pH and food go down.

Celiac disease: gluten-free-diet grains
BB-WORM

Barley
Buckwheat
Wheat
Oats
Rye
Malt

Constipation: causes
DOPED

Drugs (example: opiates)
Obstruction (examples: IBD, cancer)
Pain
Endocrine (example: hypothyroid)
Depression

Splenomegaly: causes
HICCUPS

Hematological
Infective: Kala azar, malaria, enteric fever
Congestive: constrictive pericarditis, IVC thrombosis, hepatic vein
    thrombosis, portal vein thrombosis, and splenic vein thrombosis
Collagen diseases: SLE, Felty's syndrome
Unknown etiology: tropical splenomegaly
Primary malignancies (secondaries are rare)
Storage diseases: Gaucher's disease, Niemann-Pick

Ileus: causes
MD PR GUESS

Mesenteric ischemia
Drugs (Aluminum hydroxide, Ca carbonate, opiates,
    TCA, verapamil)
Peritonitis/**P**ancreatitis (sentinel loop)
Retroperitoneal bleed or hematoma
Gram-negative sepsis
Unresolved mechanical obstruction (examples: mass,
    intussusception, blockage)
Electrolyte imbalance (example: hypokalemia)
Surgical (postoperative)
Spinal or pelvic fracture

Hematology

Anemia: non-megaloblastic causes of macrocytic anemia
HAND LAMP
Hypothyroidism
Aplastic anemia
Neonates
Drugs
Liver disease
Alcohol
Myelodysplasia
Pregnancy

Lead poisoning (chronic): features
ABCDEFGHI
Anemia/**A**norexia/**A**rthralgia/**A**bortion/**A**trophy of optic nerve
Basophilic stippling of RBC (punctate basophilia)/
  Burtonian line on gums
Colic/**C**onstipation/**C**erebral edema
Drop (wrist, foot)
Encephalopathy/**E**maciation
Foul smell of breath/**F**ailure of kidneys/**F**anconi syndrome
Gonadal dysfunction/**G**out-like picture
High BP/**H**eadache/**H**allucination/**H**yperesthesia
Impotence/**I**nsomnia/**I**rritability

Macrocytic anemia: causes
ABCDEF
Alcohol + liver disease
B$_{12}$ deficiency
Compensatory reticulocytosis (blood loss and hemolysis)
Drug (cytotoxic and AZT)/**D**ysplasia (marrow problems)
Endocrine (hypothyroidism)
Folate deficiency/**F**etus (pregnancy)

Sickle cell disease: complications
SICKLE

Strokes/**S**welling of hands and feet/**S**pleen problems
Infections/**I**nfarctions
Crises (painful, sequestration, aplastic)/**C**holelithiasis/**C**hest
   syndrome/**C**hronic hemolysis/**C**ardiac problems
Kidney disease
Liver disease/**L**ung problems
Erection (priapism)/**E**ye problems (retinopathy)

Pancytopenia: differential
All Of My Blood Has Taken Some Poison.

Aplastic anemias
Overwhelming sepsis
Megaloblastic anemias
Bone marrow infiltration
Hypersplenism
TB
SLE
Paroxysmal nocturnal hemoglobinuria

Thrombocytopenia: causes
SHAPIRO

Splenectomy
Hodgkin's disease
Arteritis
Polycythemia
Infection
Rheumatoid
Occult malignancy

Polycythemia Rubra Vera (PRV): common symptoms
PRV

Plethora/**P**ruritus
Ringing in ears
Visual blurriness

History and Physical

Sign versus symptom
sIgn:
Something **I** can detect even if patient is unconscious.
sYMptom:
Symptom is something only h**YM** knows about.

Patient examination organization
SOAP
Subjective: what the patient says
Objective: what the examiner observes
Assessment: what the examiner thinks is going on
Plan: what they intend to do about it

Pain history checklist
OPQRSTU
Onset of pain (time, duration)
Precipitating factors for pain
Quality of pain (examples: throbbing, stabbing, dull)
Region of body affected/**R**adiation/**R**elieving factors
Severity of pain (usually scale of 1–10)
Timing of pain (examples: after exercise, in evening)/
  Treatments tried
U: How does it affect U in your daily life?

Physical examination for "lumps and bumps"
6 Students and 3 Teachers go for a CAMPFIRE
Site, **S**ize, **S**hape, **S**urface, **S**kin, **S**car
Tenderness, **T**emperature, **T**ransillumination
Consistency
Attachment
Mobility
Pulsation
Fluctuation
Irreducibility
Regional lymph nodes
Edge

Patient profile (PP)
LADDERS

Living situation/**L**ifestyle
Anxiety
Depression
Daily activities (describe a typical day)
Environmental risks/**E**xposure
Relationships
Support system/**S**tress

Alcohol abuse screening questions
CAGE

1. Ever felt it necessary to **C**ut down on drinking?
2. Has anyone ever said they felt **A**nnoyed by your drinking?
3. Ever felt **G**uilty about drinking?
4. Ever felt a need to have a morning drink as an **E**ye-opener?

Family history (FH)
BALD CHASM

Blood pressure (high)
Arthritis
Lung disease
Diabetes
Cancer
Heart disease
Alcoholism
Stroke
Mental health disorders (example: depression)

Infectious Disease

Eosinophilia: differential
NAACP

Neoplasm
Allergy/**A**sthma
Addison's disease
Collagen vascular diseases
Parasites

Toxicity/Sepsis: signs
6 T's

Tachycardia
Tachypnea
Tremors
Toxic look
Tiredness
Temperature (fever)

Medications

Allopurinol: indications
STORE

Stones (history of renal stones)
Tophaceous gout (chronic)
Overproducers of urate
Renal disease
Elderly

NSAIDs: contraindications
NSAID

Nursing and pregnancy
Serious bleeding
Allergy/**A**sthma/**A**ngioedema
Impaired renal function
Drug (anticoagulant)

ACEI: contraindications
PARK

Pregnancy
Allergy
Renal artery stenosis
K increase (hyperkalemia)

Miscellaneous

Pruritus without rash: differential diagnosis
ITCHING DX
Infections (scabies, toxocariasis, etc)
Thyroidal and other endocrinopathies (diabetes mellitus)
Cancer
Hematologic diseases (iron deficiency)/**H**epatopathies/**HIV**
Idiopathic
Neurotic
Gravid (pruritus of pregnancy)
Drugs
e**X**cretory dysfunctions (uremia)

Fall: differential
I SAVED PANGS.
Illness
Syncope
Accident
Vision
Epilepsy (or other fit)
Drugs
Psychiatric (dementia)
Anemia
Neurological (Parkinson's, cerebellar, neuropathy)
Glucose (hypoglycemia)
Stroke

CT scan: indications in trauma setting
Uncle Nelson ARgues ABout Kids
Unconscious patient after head trauma
Neck injury; to confirm vertebral fracture when X-ray is equivocal
Aortic **R**upture (after X-ray, before aortogram)
ABdominal penetrating wound; when gloved finger in ER cannot determine penetration
Kidney injury leading to blood in urine; blunt abdominal trauma

ICU: management

A to Z

A: **A**sepsis/**A**irway
B: **B**ed sore/encourage **B**reathing/**B**lood pressure
C: **C**irculation/encourage **C**oughing/**C**onsciousness
D: **D**rains
E: **E**CG
F: **F**luid status
G: **G**I losses/**G**ag reflex
H: **H**ead positioning/**H**eight
I: **I**nsensible losses
J: **J**ugular venous pulse
K: **K**indness
L: **L**imb care/**L**abel
M: **M**outh care
N: **N**ociception/**N**utrition
O: **O**xygenation/**O**rient the patient
P: **P**ulse/**P**eristalsis/**P**hysiotherapy
Q: **Q**uiet surroundings
R: **R**espiratory rate/**R**estraint
S: **S**tress ulcer/**S**uctioning
T: **T**emperature
U: **U**rine
V: **V**entilator
W: **W**ounds/**W**eight
X: **X**erosis
Y: wh**Y**
Z: **Z**estful care of the patient

Musculoskeletal

Sports injuries: course of action
RICE
Rest
Ice
Compression
Elevation

Back pain: causes
DISK MASS
("Disk" suggests proximity to vertebral disc.)
Degeneration (DJD, osteoporosis, spondylosis)
Infection (UTI, PID, Pott's disease, osteomyelitis, prostatitis)/**I**njury, fracture, or compression fracture
Spondylitis (ankylosing spondyloarthropathies such as rheumatoid arthritis, Reiter's, SLE)
Kidney (stones, infarction, infection)
Multiple myeloma/**M**etastasis (from cancers of breast, kidney, lung, prostate, thyroid)
Abdominal pain (referred to the back)/**A**neurysm
Skin (herpes zoster)/**S**train/**S**coliosis and lordosis
Slipped disk/**S**pondylolisthesis

Neurology

Horner's syndrome: components
SAMPLE
Sympathetic chain injury
Anhidrosis
Miosis
Ptosis
Loss of ciliospinal reflex
Enophthalmos

Obstetrics/Gynecology

Oral contraceptive complications: warning signs
ACHES
Abdominal pain
Chest pain
Headache (severe)
Eyes (blurred vision)
Sharp leg pain

Oral contraceptives: side effects
CONTRACEPTIVES
Cholestatic jaundice
Oedema (corneal)
Nasal congestion
Thyroid dysfunction
Raised BP
Acne/**A**lopecia/**A**nemia
Cerebrovascular disease
Elevated blood sugar
Porphyria/**P**igmentation/**P**ancreatitis
Thromboembolism
Intracranial hypertension
Vomiting (progesterone only)
Erythema nodosum/**E**xtrapyramidal effects
Sensitivity to light

Breast history: checklist
LMNOP
Lump
Mammary changes
Nipple changes
Other symptoms
Patient risk factors

Breast feeding: benefits
ABCDEFGH

Infant:
Allergic condition reduced
Best food for infant
Close relationship with mother
Development of IQ, jaws, mouth

Mother:
Economical
Fitness: quick return to pre-pregnancy body shape
Guards against cancer: breast, ovary, uterus
Hemorrhage (postpartum) reduced

Breast feeding: contraindicated drugs
BREAST

Bromocriptine/**B**enzodiazepines
Radioactive isotopes/**R**izatriptan
Ergotamine/**E**thosuximide
Amiodarone/**A**mphetamines
Stimulant laxatives/**S**ex hormones
Tetracycline/**T**retinoin

Abdominal pain: causes during pregnancy
LARA CROFT

Labor
Abruption of placenta
Rupture (ectopic/uterus)
Abortion
Cholestasis
Rectus sheath hematoma
Ovarian tumor
Fibroids
Torsion of uterus

RLQ pain: brief female differential
AEIOU

Appendicitis/**A**bscess
Ectopic pregnancy/**E**ndometriosis
Inflammatory disease (pelvic)/**I**BD
Ovarian cyst (rupture, torsion)
Uteric colic/**U**rinary stones

Ovarian cancer: risk factors

Blue FILM

Breast cancer
Family history
Infertility
Low parity
Mumps

Pelvic inflammatory disease (PID): causes, effects

PID CAN be EPIC

Causes:
Chlamydia trachomatis
Actinomycetes
Neisseria gonorrhoea

Effects:
Ectopic
Pregnancy
Infertility
Chronic pain

Pelvic inflammatory disease (PID): complications

I FACE PID.

Infertility
Fitz-Hugh-Curtis syndrome
Abscess
Chronic pelvic pain
Ectopic pregnancy
Peritonitis
Intestinal obstruction
Disseminated: sepsis, endocarditis, arthritis, meninigitis

Secondary amenorrhea: causes

SOAP

Stress
OCP
Anorexia
Pregnancy

Sexual response cycle
EXPLORE

EXcitement
PLateau
Orgasmic
REsolution

Parity abbreviations (examples: G 3, P 2012)
To Peace And Love

T: of **T**erm pregnancies
P: of **P**remature births
A: of **A**bortions (spontaneous or elective)
L: of **L**ive births
(Gravida= the total number of pregnancies)

Prenatal care questions
ABCDEF

Amniotic fluid leakage?
Bleeding vaginally?
Contractions?
Dysuria?
Edema?
Fetal movement?

Alpha-fetoprotein: causes for increased maternal serum AFP during pregnancy
Increased Maternal Serum Alpha Feto Protein

Intestinal obstruction
Multiple gestation/**M**iscalculation of gestational age/**M**yeloschisis
Spina bifida cystica
Anencephaly/**A**bdominal wall defect
Fetal death
Placental abruption

Preeclampsia: classic triad
PREeclampsia

Proteinuria
Rising blood pressure
Edema

Multiple pregnancy complications
HI, PAPA

Hydramnios (Poly)
IUGR
Preterm labor
Antepartum hemorrhage
Preeclampsia
Abortion

Dysfunctional uterine bleeding (DUB): 3 major causes
DUB

Don't ovulate (anovulation: 90% of cases)
Unusual corpus luteum activity (prolonged or insufficient)
Birth control pills (since increases progesterone–estrogen ratio)

IUGR: causes
IUGR

Inherited: chromosomal and genetic disorders
Uterus: placental insufficiency
General: maternal malnutrition, smoking
Rubella and other congenital infections

Antepartum hemorrhage (APH): major differential
APH

Abruptio placentae
Placenta previa
Hemorrhage from the GU tract

Miscarriage: recurrent miscarriage causes
RIBCAGE

Radiation
Immune reaction
Bugs (infection)
Cervical incompetence
Anatomical anomaly (example: uterine septum)
Genetic (examples: aneuploidy, balanced translocation)
Endocrine

Female pelvis: shapes
GAP

In order from most to least common:
Gynecoid
Android /**A**nthropoid
Platypelloid

Labor: preterm labor causes
DISEASE

Dehydration
Infection
Sex
Exercise (strenuous)
Activities
Stress
Environmental factor

Labor: factors determining rate and outcome of labor
3 P's

Power: strength of uterine contractions
Passage: size of the pelvic inlet and outlet
Passenger: the fetus—is it big, small, have anomalies, alive or dead

Early cord clamping: indications
RAPID CS

Rh incompatibility
Asphyxia
Premature delivery
Infections
Diabetic mother
CS (caesarian section) previously

Forceps: indications for delivery
FORCEPS

Fetus alive
Os dilated
Ruptured membrane
Cervix taken up
Engagement of head
Presentation suitable
Sagittal suture in AP diameter of inlet

Fetus: cardinal movements of fetus
Don't Forget I Enjoy Really Expensive Equipment.

Descent
Flexion
Internal rotation
Extension
Restitution
External rotation
Expulsion

Delivery: instrumental delivery prerequisites
AABBCCDDEE

Analgesia
Antisepsis
Bowel empty
Bladder empty
Cephalic presentation
Consent
Dilated cervix
Disproportion
Engaged
Episiotomy

APGAR score components
SHIRT

Skin color: blue or pink
Heart rate: below 100 or over 100
Irritability (response to stimulation): none, grimace, or cry
Respirations: irregular or good
Tone (muscle): some flexion or active

Postpartum examination simplified checklist
BUBBLES

Breast
Uterus
Bowel
Bladder
Lochia
Episiotomy
Surgical site (for cesarean section)

Postpartum collapse: causes
HEPARINS

Hemorrhage
Eclampsia
Pulmonary embolism
Amniotic fluid embolism
Regional anasthetic complications
Infarction (MI)
Neurogenic shock
Septic shock

Postpartum hemorrhage (PPH): causes
4 T's

Tissue (retained placenta)
Tone (uterine atony)
Trauma (traumatic delivery, episiotomy)
Thrombin (coagulation disorders, DIC)

Postpartum hemorrhage (PPH): risk factors
PARTUM

Polyhydramnios/**P**rolonged labor/**P**revious cesarian
Antepartum hemorrhage
Recent bleeding history
Twins
Uterine fibroids
Multiparity

IUD: side effects

PAINS

Period that is late
Abdominal cramps
Increase in body temperature
Noticeable vaginal discharge
Spotting

Pediatrics

Guthrie card: diseases it identifies
Guthrie Cards Can Help Predict Bad Metabolism.

Galactosemia
Cystic fibrosis
Congenital adrenal hyperplasia
Hypothyroidism
Phenylketonuria
Biotinidase deficiency
Maple syrup urine disease

Strep throat score
NO FACE

NO cough: no cough is +1
Fever: has fever is +1
Age: less than 5 years is –1, 15–45 years is 0,
    greater than 45 years is +1
Cervical nodes: cervical nodes palpable is +1
Exudate: tonsillar exudate is +1

Scoring interpretation:
Score 0–1: no strep throat.
Score 1–3: possible strep throat, do swab test.
Score 4–5: strep throat is likely, so treat empirically.

Croup: symptoms
3 S's

Stridor
Subglottic swelling
Seal-bark cough

Ataxia-Telangiectasia (AT): common sign
AT

Absent
Thymus

VACTERL syndrome: components

VACTERL

Vertebral anomalies
Anorectal malformation
Cardiac anomaly
Tracheoesophageal fistula
Exomphalos (omphalocele)
Renal anomalies
Limb anomalies

Williams syndrome: features

WILLIAMS

Weight (low at birth, slow to gain)
Iris (stellate iris)
Long philtrum
Large mouth
Increased Ca^{++}
Aortic stenosis (and other stenoses)
Mental retardation
Swelling around eyes (periorbital puffiness)

Russell Silver syndrome: features

ABCDEF

Asymmetric limb (hemihypertrophy)
Bossing (frontal)
Clinodactyly/**C**afe-au-lait spots
Dwarf (short stature)
Excretion (GU malformation)
Face (triangular face, micrognathia)

Dentition: eruption times of permanent dentition

Mama Is In Pain; Papa Can Make Medicine.

1st **M**olar: 6 years
1st **I**ncisor: 7 years
2nd **I**ncisor: 8 years
1st **P**remolar: 9 years
2nd **P**remolar: 10 years
Canine: 11 years
2nd **M**olar: 12 years
3rd **M**olar: 18–25 years

Cyanotic congenital heart diseases
5 T's
Truncus arteriosus
Transposition of the great arteries
Tricuspid atresia
Tetralogy of Fallot
Total anomalous pulmonary venous return

Hemolytic-uremic syndrome (HUS): components
Remember to decrease the RATE of IV fluids in these patients.
Renal failure
Anemia (microangiopathic, hemolytic)
Thrombocytopenia
Encephalopathy (TTP)

Cough (chronic): differential
When cough in nursery, rock the CRADLE
Cystic fibrosis
Rings, slings, and airway things (tracheal rings)/Respiratory infections
Aspiration (swallowing dysfunction, TE fistula, gastroesophageal reflux)
Dyskinetic cilia
Lung, airway, and vascular malformations (tracheomalacia, vocal cord dysfunction)
Edema (heart failure)

Cystic fibrosis: presenting signs
CF PANCREAS
Chronic cough and wheezing
Failure to thrive
Pancreatic insufficiency (symptoms of malabsorption like steatorrhea)
Alkalosis and hypotonic dehydration
Neonatal intestinal obstruction (meconium ileus)/Nasal polyps
Clubbing of fingers/Chest radiograph with characteristic changes
Rectal prolapse
Electrolyte elevation in sweat, salty skin
Absence or congenital atresia of vas deferens
Sputum with staph or pseudomonas (mucoid)

Pyloric stenosis (congenital): presentation
3 P's

Palpable mass
Peristalsis visible
Projectile vomiting (2–4 weeks after birth)

WAGR syndrome: components
WAGR

Wilm's tumor
Aniridia
Genital abnormalities
Mental **R**etardation

Hematuria: differential in children
ABCDEFGHIJK

Anatomy (example: cysts)
Bladder (cystitis)
Cancer (Wilms tumor)
Drug-related (cyclophosphamide)
Exercise-induced
Factitious (Münchhausen by proxy)
Glomerulonephritis
Hematology (bleeding disorder, sickle cell)
Infection (UTI) /**In**Jury (trauma)
Kidney stones (hypercalciuria)

Pediatric measurements

Head circumference with age:

(Remember 3, 9, and multiples of 5)
Newborn 35 cm
3 months 40 cm
9 months 45 cm
3 years 50 cm
9 years 55 cm

Weights of children with age:

Newborn 3 kg
6 months 6 kg (2 × birth weight at 6 months)
1 year 10 kg (3 × birth weight at 1 year)
3 years 15 kg (odd years, add 5 kg until 11 years)
5 years 20 kg
7 years 25 kg
9 years 30 kg
11 years 35 kg (add 10 kg thereafter)
13 years 45 kg
15 years 55 kg
17 years 65 kg

Pediatric milestones in development

1 year

• single words

2 years

• 2-word sentences
• understands 2-step commands

3 years

• 3-word combos
• repeats 3 digits
• rides tricycle

4 years

• draws square
• counts 4 objects

Short stature: differential
ABCDEFG

Alone (neglected infant)
Bone dysplasias (rickets, scoliosis, mucopolysaccharidoses)
Chromosomal (Turner's, Down's)
Delayed growth
Endocrine (low growth hormone, Cushing's, hypothyroid)
Familial
GI malabsorption (celiac, Crohn's)

Pediatric history taking
Patient name, presenting complaint, history of presenting complaint, and past medical history, Then ask BIFIDA

Birth details and problems
Immunizations
Feeding
Infection, exposure to
Development, normality of
Allergies

Neonatal resuscitation: successive steps
Do What Pediatricians Say To, Or Be Inviting Costly Malpractice.

Drying
Warming
Positioning
Suctioning
Tactile stimulation
Oxygen
Bagging
Intubate endotracheally
Chest compressions
Medications

Beckwith-Wiedemann syndrome: features
HOMO

Hypoglycemia
Omphalocele
Macroglossia/**M**acrosomia
Organomegaly

Psychology

Mental state examination: stages in order
Assessed Mental State To Be Positively Clinically Unremarkable

Appearance and behavior (observe state, clothing...)
Mood (recent spirit)
Speech (rate, form, content)
Thinking (thoughts, perceptions)
Behavioral abnormalities
Perception abnormalities
Cognition (time, place, age...)
Understanding of condition (ideas, expectations, concerns)

Schizophrenia: negative features
4 A's

Ambivalence
Affective incongruence
Associative loosening
Autism

Biological symptoms in psychiatry
SCALED

Sleep disturbance
Concentration
Appetite
Libido
Energy
Diurnal mood variation

Depression: major episode DSM-IV criteria
SIG E CAPS
Sleep disturbance
Interest loss
Guilt (or intense worthlessness)
Energy loss
Concentration loss
Appetite changes
Psychomotor agitation or retardation
Suicidal tendency

Depression: melancholic features (DSM IV)
MELANcholic
Morning worsening of symptoms/psycho**M**otor agitation, retardation/early **M**orning wakening
Excessive guilt
Loss of emotional reactivity
ANorexia/**AN**hedonia

Dementia: main causes
VITAMIN D VEST
Vitamin deficiency (B12, folate, thiamine)
Intracranial tumor
Trauma (head injury)
Anoxia
Metabolic (diabetes)
Infection (postencephalitis, HIV)
Normal pressure hydrocephalus
Degenerative (examples: Alzheimer's, Huntington's, CJD)
Vascular (multi-infarct dementia)
Endocrine (hypothyroid)
Space-occupying lesion (chronic subdural hematoma)
Toxic (alcohol)

Mania: cardinal symptoms
DIG FAST

Distractibility
Indiscretion (DSM-IV's: the excessive involvement in pleasurable activities)
Grandiosity
Flight of ideas
Activity increase
Sleep deficit (decreased need for sleep)
Talkativeness (pressured speech)

Mania: diagnostic criteria
Must have 3 of MANIAC

Mouth (pressure of speech)/**M**ood
Activity increased
Naughty (disinhibition)
Insomnia
Attention (distractibility)
Confidence (grandiose ideas)

Hallucinations: hypnagogic versus hypnopompic definition

Hypna**GO**gic = **GO** to sleep

(Hypnagogic hallucinations arise when go to sleep, hypnopompic arise when awaken.)

Borderline personality: traits
PRAISE

Paranoid ideas
Relationship instability
Affective instability/**A**bandonment fears/**A**ngry outbursts
Impulsiveness/**I**dentity disturbance
Suicidal behavior/**S**elf-harming behavior
Emptiness

Cluster personality disorders

Cluster A Disorder = **A**typical (unusual and eccentric)
Cluster B Disorder = **B**east (uncontrolled wildness)
Cluster C Disorder = **C**oward (avoidant type), **C**ompulsive
   (obsessive-compulsive type), or **C**lingy (dependent type)

Sleep stages: features

DElta waves during **DE**epest sleep (stages 3 and 4, slow-wave)
d**REaM** during **REM** sleep

REM: features

REM
Rapid pulse/**R**espiratory rate
Erection
Mental activity increase/**M**uscle paralysis

Narcolepsy: symptoms, epidemiology

CHAP (usually seen in a young male, or "chap")
Cataplexy
Hallucinations
Attacks of sleep
Paralysis on waking

AIDS dementia complex (ADC): features

AIDS
Atrophy of cortex
Infection/**I**nflammation
Demyelination
Six months death

Autistic disorder: features
AUTISTICS

Again and again (repetitive behavior)
Unusual abilities
Talking (language) delay
IQ subnormal
Social development poor
Three years onset
Inherited component (35% concordance)
Cognitive impairment
Self injury

Kübler-Ross dying process: stages
Death Always Brings Great Acceptance.

Denial
Anger
Bargaining
Grieving
Acceptance

Renal

Non-gap acidosis: causes
HARD UP
Hyperalimentation
Acetazolamide (carbonic anhydrase inhibitors)
RTA
Diarrhea
Ureterosigmoidostomy
Pancreatic fistula

Metabolic acidosis: causes
KUSSMAL
Ketoacidosis
Uremia
Sepsis
Salicylates
Methanol
Alcohol
Lactic acidosis

Anion gap metabolic acidosis: causes
MUDPILES
Methanol
Uremia
Diabetic ketoacidosis
Paraldehyde
Infection
Lactic acidosis
Ethylene glycol
Salicylates

Renal failure (acute): management
Manage AEIOU
Anemia/**A**cidosis
Electrolytes and fluids
Infections
Other measures (examples: nutrition, nausea, vomiting)
Uremia

Dialysis: indications
HAVE PEE

Hyperkalemia (refractory)
Acidosis (refractory)
Volume overload
Elevated BUN (>36 mM)
Pericarditis
Encephalopathy
Edema (pulmonary)

Tumors of renal pelvis: indications
Bilateral is SUPER.

Stenosis of the urethra
Urethral valve
Prostatic enlargement
Extensive bladder tumor
Retroperitoneal fibrosis

Enlarged kidneys: causes
SHAPE

Scleroderma
HIV nephropathy
Amyloidosis
Polycystic kidney disease
Endocrinopathy (diabetes)

Glomerular disease with reduced complement level
PELICAN

Post-streptococcal glomerulonephritis
Endocarditis (subacute)
Lupus erythematosus
Idiopathic membranoproliferative glomerulonephritis
Cryoglobulinemia
Abscess (visceral)
Nephritis

Urinary incontinence: differential
DIAPERS

Delirium
Infection
Atrophic urethritis and vaginitis
Pharmaceuticals/**P**sychologic
Excessive urine output
Restricted mobility
Stool impaction

Hematuria: differential
HEMATURIA

Hereditary (PCK and OWR)/**H**enoch-Schönlein purpura
Embolism (infective endocarditis)
Malignant HTN
Acute and chronic glomerulonephritis/Ig**A** nephropathy
Tumors/**T**rauma/**T**oxic drugs
Urolithiasis
Renal papillary necrosis
Infection (pyelonephritis, cystitis, urethritis)
Anticoagulants

Nephrectomy: indications
4 T's

Trauma
Tumor
TB
Transplantation

Reproductive

Epididymitis: bacterial causes
CENT

Chlamydia trachomatis
E. coli
Neisseria gonorrhea
Tuberculosis bacteria

Prostatism: initial symptoms
FUN

Frequency
Urgency
Nocturia

Impotence: causes
PLANE

Psychogenic: performance anxiety
Libido: decreased with androgen deficiency, drugs
Autonomic neuropathy: impede blood flow redirection
Nitric oxide deficiency: impaired synthesis, decreased blood
    pressure
Erectile reserve: cannot maintain an erection

Male erectile dysfunction (MED): biological causes
MED

Medicines (examples: propranolol, methyldopa, SSRI)
Ethanol
Diabetes mellitus

Premature ejaculation: treatment
2 S's

SSRIs (fluoxetine)
Squeezing technique (glans pressure before climax)

Respiratory

Auscultation: crackles (rales)
PEBbles

Pneumonia
Edema of lung
Bronchitis

Acute stridor: differential
ABCDEFGH

With fever:
Abscess
Bacterial tracheitis
Croup
Diphtheria
Epiglottitis

Without fever:
Foreign body
Gas (Toxic Gas)
Hypersensitivity

Clubbing: respiratory causes
ABCDEF

Abscess (lung)
Bronchiectasis (including CF)
Cancer (lung)
Decreased oxygen (hypoxia)
Empyema
Fibrosing alveolitis

Chronic cough: full differential
gASPS AND COUGH

Asthma
Smoking, chronic bronchitis
Post-infection
Sinusitis, post-nasal drip
ACE inhibitor
Neoplasm
Diverticulum
Congestive heart failure
Outer ear
Upper airway obstruction
GI-airway fistula
Hypersensitivity

Wheezing: causes
ASTHMA

Asthma
Small airways disease
Tracheal obstruction
Heart failure
Mastocytosis or carcinoid
Anaphylaxis or allergy

Asthma: precipitating factors for acute attack
DIPLOMAT

Drugs (examples: aspirin, NSAIDs, beta-blockers)
Infections (URI/LRI)
Pollutants (at home, at work)
Laughter (emotion)
Oesophageal reflux (nocturnal asthma)
Mites
Activity and exercise
Temperature (cold)

Bronchiectasis: differential diagnosis
BRONCHIECTASIS
Bronchial cyst
Repeated gastric acid aspiration
Or due to foreign bodies
Necrotizing pneumonia
Chemical corrosive substances
Hypogammaglobulinemia
Immotile cilia syndrome
Eosinophilia (pulmonary)
Cystic fibrosis
Tuberculosis (primary)
Atopic bronchial asthma
Streptococcal pneumonia
In Young's syndrome
Staphylococcal pneumonia

Pulmonary edema: treatment
LMNOP
Lasix
Morphine
Nitrates (NTG)
Oxygen
Position (upright versus flat)

Pulmonary fibrosis: causes
SCAR
Upper lobe:
Silicosis/**S**arcoidosis
Coal worker pneumonoconiosis
Ankylosing spondylitis
Radiation

Lower lobe:
Systemic sclerosis
Cryptogenic fibrosing alveolitis
Asbestosis
Rheumatoid arthritis

Pulmonary fibrosis: drug-causing pulmonary fibrosis
BBAT

Busulfan
Bleomycin
Amiodarone
Tocainide

Pleural effusion: investigations
PLEURA

Pleural fluid (thoracentesis)
Lung, pleural biopsy
ESR
Ultrasound
Radiogram
Analysis of blood

Pneumonia: risk factors
INSPIRATION

Immunosuppression
Neoplasia
Secretion retention
Pulmonary edema
Impaired alveolar macrophages
Responsiveness to intervention (prior)
Antibiotics and cytotoxics
Tracheal instrumentation
IV dug abuse
Other (general debility, immobility)
Neurologic impairment of cough reflex (NMJ disorders)

Caplan syndrome: characteristics
CAPlan

Coal-worker pneumoconiosis
Arthritis
Pulmonary nodule

Surgery

Scrotum swelling: differential
THE THEATRES

Torsion
Hernia
Epididymitis, orchitis
Trauma
Hydrocele, varicocele, hematoma
Edema
Appendix testes (torsion, hemorrhage)
Tumor
Recurrent leukemia
Epididymal cyst
Syphilis, TB

Testicular atrophy: differential
TESTES SHRINK

Trauma
Exhaustional atrophy
Sequelae
Too little food
Elderly
Semen obstruction
Sex hormone therapy
Hypopituitarism
Radiation
Inflammatory orchitis
Not descended
Klinefelter's

Edema causes: localized
ALIVE

Allergic (angioedema)
Lymphatic (elephantiasis)
Inflammatory (infection, injury)
VEnous (DVT, chronic venous insufficiency)

Esophageal cancer risk factors
PC BASTARDS

Plummer-Vinson syndrome
Celiac disease
Barrett's
Alcohol
Smoking
Tylosis
Achalasia
Russia (geographical distribution)
Diet
Stricture

Abdomen: inspection
5 S's

Size
Shape
Scars
Skin lesions
Stoma

GI bleeding: causes
ABCDEFGHI

Angiodysplasia
Bowel cancer
Colitis
Diverticulitis/**D**uodenal ulcer
Epistaxis/**E**sophageal (cancer, esophagitis, varices)
Fistula (anal, aortoenteric)
Gastric (cancer, ulcer, gastritis)
Hemorrhoids
Infectious diarrhea/**I**BD/**I**schemic bowel

Medical Reference Guide

Appendectomy: complications
WRAP IF HOT.
Wound infection
Respiratory (atelectasis, pneumonia)
Abscess (pelvic)
Portal pyemia
Ileus (paralytic)
Fecal fistula
Hernia (right inguinal)
Obstruction (intestinal due to adhesions)
Thrombus (DVT)

Hernias of abdominal wall
Think of the abdomen as a PAIL.
These are the four groups of hernias.
Pelvic hernias: obturator, perineal, sciatic
Anterior hernias: epigastric, incisional, Spigelian, supravesical, umbilical
Inguinal hernias: indirect, direct, femoral
Lumbar hernias: inferior lumbar triangle (Petit), superior lumbar triangle (Grynfelt)

Inguinal mass: differential
Hernias Like To Swell Very Much.
Hernias (inguinal, femoral)
Lymph nodes
Testicle (ectopic, undescended)
Spermatic cord (lipoma, hydrocele)
Vascular (femoral aneurysm, saphenous varix)
Muscle (psoas abscess)

Melanoma sites
SEA
Melanoma sites, in order of frequency:
Skin
Eyes
Anus

224

Fistulas: conditions preventing closure
FRIEND

Foreign body
Radiation
Infection/**In**flammation (Crohn's)
Epithelialization
Neoplasia
Distal obstruction

Compartment syndrome: signs and symptoms
6 P's

Pain
Pallor
Pulseless
Paresthesia
Pressure (increased)
Poikilothermia

Disease description: organization of answer
In A Surgeon's Gown, Physicians May Make Some Clinical Progress.

Incidence
Age
Sex
Geography
Predisposing factors
Macroscopic appearance
Microscopic appearance
Spread
Clinical features
Prognosis

Hematocele: etiology
3T's and 2 H's

Tumor
Torsion
Trauma
Hydrocele as a complication
Hemophilia (blood diseases)

Varicose veins: symptoms
AEIOU

Aching
Eczema
Itching
Oedema
Ulceration (LDS, hemosiderin, varicosities)

Swollen leg: unilateral swelling causes
TV BAIL

Trauma
Venous (varicose veins, DVT, venous insufficiency)
Baker's cyst
Allergy
Inflammation (cellulitis)
Lymphedema

Ulcers: edge types
F PURE

Flat (example: venous)
Punched-out (examples: trophic, arterial)
Undetermined (examples: pressure, TB)
Rolled (example: Basal Cell Carcinoma)
Everted (example: Small Cell Carcinoma)

Postoperative complications (immediate)
Post-op PROBS

Pain
Primary hemorrhage
Reactionary hemorrhage
Oliguria
Basal atelectasis
Shock/**S**epsis

Postoperative fever causes
6 W's

Wind: pulmonary system is primary source of fever over first
48 hours, may have pneumonia
Wound: infection at surgical site
Water: check IV for phlebitis
Walk: deep venous thrombosis, due to pelvic pooling or restricted
mobility related to pain and fatigue
Whiz: urinary tract infection if urinary catheterization
Wonder drugs: drug-induced fever

Postoperative order list checkup
FLAVOR

Fluids
Laboratories
Activity
Vital signs
Oral allowances
Rx (medications)

TPN indications
MISIPPI Burning

Major visceral injury
IBD
Sepsis
Ileus
Post-op
Paralysis
Intestinal fistula
Burns

Vasculitis

Behçet's syndrome: diagnostic criteria
PROSE

Pathergy test (i/d saline injection)
Recurrent genital ulceration
Oral ulceration (recurrent)
Skin lesions
Eye lesions

Oral ulceration is central criteria, plus any 2 others.

Raynaud's disease: causes
BAD CT

Blood disorders (polycythemia)
Arterial (atherosclerosis, Buerger's)
Drugs (beta-blockers)
Connective tissue disorders (rheumatoid arthritis, SLE)
Traumatic (vibration injury)

SLE: factors making SLE active
UV PRISM

UV (sunshine)
Pregnancy
Reduced drug (steroid)
Infection
Stress
More drug

CREST syndrome: variant of scleroderma
CREST

Calcinosis
Raynaud's
Esophageal dysfunction
Sclerodactyly
Telangiectasias

Common
Medical
Abbreviations

Explanatory Notes

The list is in alphabetical order of abbreviations, not of definitions.

Any abbreviation beginning with a number will be alphabetized according to the first letter following the number. If the abbreviation is only numbers, such as 2/2, then it will be alphabetized according to its definition.

Some abbreviations represent more than one definition. If so, the multiple definitions will appear directly below each other and the abbreviation itself will not repeat, unless the abbreviation is color-coded differently. (See below for color-coding key.)

The three different colors used throughout the list represent the following:

> **Black** = General/all specialties
>
> **Blue** = OB/GYN-specific abbreviations
>
> **Red** = Psychology-specific abbreviations

A

A-a	Alveolar-arterial gradient
AA	Alcoholics Anonymous
	African American
AAA	Abdominal aortic aneurysm
AAD	Antibiotic-associated diarrhea
AAO	Alert and oriented
AAS	Acute abdominal series
AAT	Activity as tolerated
AB	Antibody
Ab	Abortion (includes elective, therapeutic, and miscarriages)
ABCD	Airway, breathing, circulation, disability
ABCs	Airway, breathing, circulation
ABD	Abdomen
ABDO	Abdominal
ABG	Arterial blood gas
ABI	Ankle brachial index
	Acquired brain injury
ABO	Landsteiner's blood grouping system
ABPA	Allergic bronchopulmonary aspergillosis
Abx	Antibiotics
AC	Anterior chamber
	Acromioclavicular
	Ante cibum (before meals)
ACA	Anterior cerebral artery
ACE-I	Angiotensin-converting enzyme inhibitor
ACL	Anterior cruciate ligament
ACLS	Advanced cardiac life support
ACS	Acute coronary syndrome
ACTH	Adrenocorticotropic hormone
ad lib	Ad libitum (as needed or desired)
ADA	American Diabetes Association
ADD	Attention deficit disorder
ADE	Adverse drug effect
ADH	Antidiuretic hormone
ADHD	Attention deficit hyperactivity disorder
ADL	Activities of daily living
ADR	Acute dystonic reaction
	Adverse drug reaction
AE	Above elbow
AEA	Above-elbow amputation
AED	Antiepileptic drug
	Automatic external defibrillator
AF	Atrial fibrillation

Medical Reference Guide

AFB	Acid-fast bacilli
AFI	Amniotic fluid index
AFL	Atrial flutter
AFP	Alpha-fetoprotein
AFVSS	Afebrile vital signs stable
A/G	Albumin/globulin ratio
AH	Auditory hallucinations
AI	Aortic insufficiency
AIDS	Acquired immune deficiency syndrome
AIN	Acute interstitial nephritis
AK	Above knee
	Actinic keratosis
AKA	Above-knee amputation
alk phos	Alkaline phosphatase
ALL	Acute leukemia
	Allergies
ALP	Alkaline phosphatase
ALS	Advanced life support
	Amyotrophic lateral sclerosis
ALT	Alanine aminotransferase
AMA	Advanced maternal age
	Against medical advice
	American Medical Association
amb	Ambulate
AMD	Aging macular degeneration
AMI	Acute myocardial infarction
	Anterior myocardial infarction
AML	Acute myelogenous leukemia
Amnio	Amniocentesis
AMS	Acute mountain sickness
	Altered mental status
ANA	Antinuclear antibody
ANC	Absolute neutrophil count
AND	Axillary node dissection
ANF	Antinuclear factor
Angio	Angiography
ANS	Autonomic nervous system
ante	Before
AOB	Alcohol on breath
AODM	Adult-onset diabetes mellitus
AP	Abdominal-perineal
	Anteroposterior
A/P	Assessment and plan
APC	Atrial premature contraction
APD	Afferent pupillary defect
APGAR	Appearance, pulse, grimace, activity, respiratory

APPY	Appendectomy
APS	Adult Protective Services
ARB	Angiotensin receptor blocker
ARDS	Adult respiratory distress syndrome
ARF	Acute renal failure
AROM	Artificial rupture of membranes
AS	Aortic stenosis
ASA	Acetylsalicylic acid
ASCVD	Atherosclerotic cardiovascular disease
ASD	Atrial septal defect
ASHD	Atherosclerotic heart disease
ASO	Anti-streptolysin-O titer
AST	Aspartate aminotransferase
ASU	Ambulatory surgery unit
ATN	Acute tubular necrosis
AV	Aortic valve
	Atrioventricular
A/V Nicking	Arteriolar/venous nicking
A/V Ratio	Arteriolar/venous ratio
AVF	Arteriovenous fistula
AVM	Arteriovenous malformation
AVN	Atrionentricular
	Avascular necrosis
AVNRT	Atrioventricular nodal reentrant tachycardia
AVR	Aortic valve replacement
AVSS	Afebrile, vital signs stable
AXR	Abdominal X-ray
AZT	Zidovudine

B

B	Bilateral
BAE	Barium enema
BBB	Bundle branch block
BBOW	Bulging bag of water
BBT .	Basal body temperature
BC	Bone conduction
BCC	Basal cell carcinoma
BCG	Bacille Calmette-Guérin
BCPs	Birth control pills
BDR	Background diabetic retinopathy
BE	Bacterial endocarditis
	Barium
BEE	Basal energy expenditure
BET	Benign essential tremor

BID	Bis in die (twice a day)
BIPAP	Bi-level positive airway pressure
ß-hCG	ß-human chorionic gonadotropin
BK	Below knee
BKA	Below-knee amputation
bili	Bilirubin
bili T/D	Bilirubin total and direct
BL CX	Blood culture
BM	Bone marrow
	Bowel movement
BMD	Bone mineral density
BMI	Body mass index
BMR	Basal metabolic rate
BMT	Bone marrow transplant
BOW	Bag of water
BP	Blood pressure
BPD	Bipolar disorder
	Borderline personality disorder
BPD	Bronchopulmonary dysplasia
BPD	Biparietal diameter
BPH	Benign prostate hypertrophy
BPM	Beats per minute
BPP	Biophysical profile
BPV	Benign positional vertigo
BR	Bed rest
BRAO	Branch retinal artery occlusion
BRB	Bright-red blood
BRBPR	Bright-red blood per rectum
BRF	Breast feeding
BRP	Bathroom privileges
BRVO	Branch retinal vein occlusion
BS	Bowel sounds
	Breath sounds
BSA	Body surface area
BSO	Bilateral salpingo-oophorectomy
BSU	Bartholin's, Skene's, urethra
BTBV	Beat-to-beat variability
BTL	Bilateral tubal ligation
BUN	Blood urea nitrogen
BW	Body weight
BX	Biopsy

C

C/	With

Common Medical Abbreviations

CA	Cancer
CAA	Crystalline amino acids
CABG	Coronary artery bypass graft
CAD	Coronary artery disease
CAP	Community-acquired pneumonia
CARDS	Cardiology
CAT	Cataract
	Computerized axial tomography
CATH	Catheterization
CB	Cerebellar
C/B	Complicated by
CBC	Complete blood count
CBD	Closed bag drainage
	Common bile duct
CBI	Continuous bladder irrigation
CBR	Chronic bed rest
cc	Cubic centimeter
CC	Chief complaint
CCC	Central corneal clouding
CCK	Cholycystectomy
CCU	Cardiac care unit
	Clean catch urine
CCV	Critical closing volume
C/D/I	Clean/dry/intact
C DIF	*Clostridium difficile*
CE	Cervical examination
CEA	Carcinoembryonic antigen
CF	Cystic fibrosis
CGL	Chronic granulocytic leukemia
Chem Dep	Chemical dependency
CHF	Congestive heart failure
CHI	Closed head injury
CHO	Carbohydrate
chol	Cholesterol
CI	Cardiac index
	Confidence interval
CIC	Clean intermittent catheterization
CIDP	Chronic inflammatory demyelinating polyneuropathy
CIN	Cervical intraepithelial neoplasia
CK	Creatinine kinase
CL	Chloride
CLL	Chronic lymphocytic leukemia
CM	Cardiomegaly
CML	Chronic myelogenous leukemia
CMP	Cardiomyopathy
CMR	Chief medical resident

CMT	Cervical motion tenderness
CMV	Cytomegalovirus
CN	Cranial nerves
CNIS	Carotid non-invasive study
CNS	Central nervous system
COPD	Chronic obstructive pulmonary disease
CO	Carbon monoxide
	Cardiac output
C/O	Complains of
CO_2	Carbon dioxide
COLD	Chronic obstructive lung disease
CP	Carotid pulse
	Cerebral palsy
CPAP	Continuous positive airway pressure
CPD	Cephalopelvic disproportion
CPK	Creatine phosphokinase
CPP	Cerebral perfusion pressure
CPPD	Calcium pyrophosphate disease
CPR	Cardiopulmonary resuscitation
CPS	Child Protective Services
CPU	Chest pain unit
CRAO	Central retinal artery occlusion
CRCL	Creatinine clearance
creat	Creatinine
CRF	Chronic renal failure
CRFs	Cardiac risk factors
CRH	Corticotrophin-releasing hormone
CRI	Chronic renal insufficiency
CRL	Crown-rump length
CRP	C-reactive protein
CRVO	Central retinal vein occlusion
C/S	Cesarean section
C&S	Culture and sensitivity
C-section	Cesarean section
CSF	Cerebral spinal fluid
	Cerebrospinal fluid
CST	Contraction stress test
CT	*Chlamydia trachomatis*
	Computerized tomography
CTA	Clear to auscultation
Ctx	Contractions
CVA	Cerebrovascular accident
	Costovertebral angle
CVL	Central venous line
CVP	Central venous pressure
CVS	Cardiovascular system

CVS	Chorionic villus sampling
C/W	Compared with
	Consistent with
Cx	Cervix
CX	Culture
CXR	Chest X-ray

D

D	Diarrhea
DAT	Diet as tolerated
DAW	Dispense as written
DB	Direct bilirubin
DBP	Diastolic blood pressure
DC	Diffusing capacity
	Discharge
	Discontinue
	Doctor of chiropractics
d/c	Discharge
	Discontinue
D&C	Dilation and curettage
DCIS	Ductal carcinoma in situ
DDAVP	Desmopressin acetate
DDX	Differential diagnosis
D&E	Dilatation and extraction
DF	Dorsiflexion
DFA	Direct fluorescent antibody
DFE	Dilated fundus examination
DGI	Disseminated gonococcal infection
DI	Detrusor instability
	Diabetes insipidus
DI	Diamniotic twins
	Dichorionic twins
DIC	Disseminated intravascular coagulopathy
DIF	Differential
DIGFAST	Sx of mania: distractibility, insomnia, grandiosity, flight of ideas, appetite (increase or decrease), speech (pressured), thoughtlessness
Dig level	Digoxin level
DIP	Distal interphalangeal (joint)
DJD	Degenerative joint disease
DKA	Diabetic ketoacidosis
dL	Deciliter
DLco	Carbon monoxide diffusing capacity
DM	Diabetes mellitus

DNI	Do not intubate
DNR	Do not resuscitate
DO	Doctor of osteopathy
D/O	Disorder
DO$_2$	Oxygen diffusion
DOA	Dead on arrival
DOB	Date of birth
DOE	Dyspnea on exertion
DOT	Directly observed therapy
DOU	Direct observation unit
DP	Dorsalis pedis
DPL	Diagnostic peritoneal lavage
DPOA	Durable Power of Attorney
DPTP	Diphtheria, pertussis, tetanus, polio
DRE	Digital rectal examination
D/T	Due to
DTR	Deep tendon reflex
DTs	Delirium tremens
DU	Duodenal ulcer
DVT	Deep venous thrombosis
D5W	Dextrose 5% in water
Dx	Diagnosis

E

E	Estrogen
E3	Estriol
EAA	Essential amino acids
EAb	Elective abortion
EBL	Estimated blood loss
EBM	Evidence-based medicine
EBRT	External beam radiation therapy
EBV	Epstein-Barr virus
ECG	Electrocardiogram
ECHO	Echocardiogram
ECMO	Extra-corporeal membrane oxygenation
ECT	Electro-convulsive therapy
ED	Erectile dysfunction
EDD	Estimated date of delivery
EDC	Estimated date of confinement
EDL	Extensor digitorum longus
EEG	Electroencephalogram
EF	Ejection fraction (in reference to ventricular function)
EFAD	Essential fatty acid deficiency
EFM	Electronic fetal monitoring

EFW	Estimated fetal weight
EGA	Estimated gestational age
EGD	Esophago-gastro-duodenoscopy
EHL	Extensor hallucis longus
EIC	Epidermal inclusion cyst
EJ	External jugular
EKG	Electrocardiogram
ELF	Elective low forceps
EM	Electron microscopy
EMB	Endometrial biopsy
EMG	Electromyelogram
EMS	Emergency Medical System
EMT	Emergency medical technician
EMV	Eyes, motor, verbal response (Glasgow coma scale)
ENT	Ears, nose, throat
E/O	Evidence of
EOM	Extraocular muscles
EOMI	Extraocular muscles intact
Eos	Eosinophils
EPO	Erythropoietin
EPS	Electrophysiologic study
ER	Emergency room
	External Rotation
ERCP	Endoscopic retrograde cholangio-pancreotography
ERT	Estrogen replacement therapy
ES	Epidural steroids
ESI	Epidural steroid injection
ESLD	End-stage liver disease
ESR	Erythrocyte sedimentation rate
ESRD	End-stage renal disease
ESWL	Extracorporeal shock wave lithotripsy
ET	Endotracheal
EtOH	Ethanol
ETT	Endotracheal tube
	Exercise tolerance test
EUA	Examination under anesthesia
EWCL	Extended-wear contact lens
EX LAP	Exploratory laparotomy
EX FIX	External fixation
EXT	Extremities

F

FA	Fluorescent antibody
FAVD	Forceps-assisted vaginal delivery

FB	Foreign body
F/B	Followed by
FBS	Fasting blood sugar
FDP	Fibrin degradation product
Fe	Iron
FEF25-75	Maximum mid-expiratory flow
FEM	Femoral
FENA	Fractional excretion of sodium
FEV$_1$	Forced expiratory volume within 1 second
FF	Fundus firm
FF@U	Fundus firm at umbilicus
FFP	Fresh frozen plasma
FH	Fundal height
FHR	Fetal heart rate
FHT	Fetal heart tracing
fib	Fibrinogen
FL	Femur length
Flex Sig	Flexible sigmoidoscopy
FLM	Fetal lung maturity
FM	Fetal movement
FMI	Fetal movement index
F&N	Febrile and neutropenic
FNA	Fine-needle aspirate
FOBT	Fetal occult blood testing
FOS	Force of stream
	Full of stool
FP	Family practitioner
FRC	Functional residual capacity
FSE	Fetal scalp electrode
FSG	Fingerstick glucose
FSH	Follicle-stimulating hormone
FT	Full term
FTP	Failure to progress
FTT	Failure to thrive
F/U	Follow-up
FUO	Fever of unknown origin
FVC	Forced vital capacity
FWB	Fetal well-being
FX	Fracture

G

g	Grams
G	Gravida
	Guaiac (followed by + or −)

Common Medical Abbreviations

GA	Gestational age
GA	General anesthesia
GAD	Generalized anxiety disorder
GAS	Group A *streptococcus*
	Guaiac all stools
GB	Gallbladder
GBM	Glioblastoma multiforme
GBS	Group B streptococcus
	Guillain-Barré syndrome
GC	Gonococcus
	Gonorrhea
GCS	Glasgow coma scale
GCSF	Granulocyte colony-stimulating factor
GDM	Gestational diabetes mellitus
GERD	Gastroesophageal reflux disease
GERI	Geriatrics
GET	General endotracheal
GETA	General endotracheal anesthesia
GETT	General by endotracheal tube
GFR	Glomerular filtration rate
GGT	Gamma glutamly transferase
GH	Growth hormone
GI	Gastrointestinal
GIB	Gastrointestinal bleeding
GIFT	Gamete intra-fallopian tube transfer
GLC	Glaucoma
glu	Glucose
GMR	Gallups, murmurs, rubs
GN	Glomerulonephritis
GNR	Gram-negative rod
GnRH	Gonadotropin-releasing hormone
GOO	Gastric outlet obstruction
G#P#	Gravida (number of pregnancies); see also Para
GPC	Gram-positive coccus
GS	Gram stain
GSW	Gunshot wound
GTD	Gestational trophoblastic disease
GTT	Glucose tolerance test
G-Tube	Gastric feeding tube
GU	Gastric ulcer
	Genitourinary
GVHD	Graft versus host disease
GXT	Graded exercise tolerance (stress test)

H

H/A	Headache
HAART	Highly active antiretroviral therapy
HACE	High-altitude cerebral edema
HAPE	High-altitude pulmonary edema
HAV	Hepatitis A virus
Hb	Hemoglobin
HBsAg	Hepatitis B surface antigen
HBV	Hepatitis B virus
HCC	Hepatocellular carcinoma
HCG	Human chorionic gonadotropin
HCL	Hard contact lens
HCM	Health care maintenance
HCT	Hematocrit
HCV	Hepatitis C virus
HD	Hemodialysis
	Huntington's disease
HDL	High-density lipoprotein
HEENT	Head, eyes, ears, nose, throat
HELLP	Hemolysis, elevated liver tests, and low platelets
HEME/ONC	Hematology/oncology
Hg	Mercury
HgB	Hemoglobin
HGH	Human growth hormone
HGSIL	High-grade squamous intraepithelial lesion
HH	Hiatal hernia
H&H	Hemoglobin and hematocrit
HI	Homicidal ideation
5-HIAA	5-hydroxyindoleacetic acid
Hib	*Hemophilus* influenza B
HIT	Heparin-induced thrombocytopenia
HIV	Human immunodeficiency virus
HJR	Hepatojugular reflex
HL	Heparin lock
H/O	History of
HOB	Head of bed
HOCM	Hypertrophic obstructive cardiomyopathy
HOH	Hard of hearing
HONK	Hyperosmolar non-ketotic state
HPF	High-power field (microscopy)
HPI	History of present illness
HPL	Human placental lactogen
HPV	Human Papillomavirus
HR	Heart rate
HRT	Hormone replacement therapy

HS	Hora somni (bedtime, hour of sleep)
HSG	Hysterosalpingogram
HSM	Hepatosplenomegaly
	Holosystolic murmur
HSP	Henoch-Schönlein purpura
HSV	Herpes simplex virus
HTN	Hypertension
HU	Holding unit
HUS	Hemolytic uremic syndrome
Hx	History

I

I+	With ionic contrast (in reference to a CAT scan)
I–	Without ionic contrast (in reference to a CAT scan)
IA	Intra-articular
IABP	Intra-aortic balloon pump
IADL	Instrumental activities of daily living
IBD	Inflammatory bowel disease
IBS	Irritable bowel syndrome
IBW	Ideal body weight
ICA	Internal carotid artery
ICD	Implantable cardiac defibrillator
ICH	Intracranial hemorrhage
ICP	Intracranial pressure
ICS	Intercostal space
ICSI	Intracytoplasmic sperm injection
ID	Identifying data
	Infectious disease
I&D	Incise and drain
IDDM	Insulin-dependent diabetes mellitus
IDL	Intermediate density lipoprotein
IE	Infective endocarditis
	Inspiratory effort
IFN	Interferon
IG	Immunoglobulin
IH	Inguinal hernia (usually preceded by L or R)
IHSS	Insulin-dependent diabetes mellitus
IJ	Internal jugular
IL	Indirect laryngoscopy
	Interleukin
ILD	Interstitial lung disease
ILF	Indicated low forceps
IM	Intramuscular
IMF	Indicated mid forceps

IMI	Inferior myocardial infarction
IMP	Impression
IMV	Intermittent mandatory ventilation
INF	Intravenous nutritional fluid
INR	International normalization ratio
I&O	Ins and outs
IOL	Intraocular lens
IOP	Intraocular pressure
IP	Interphalangeal (joint)
IPPB	Intermittent positive pressure breathing
IPF	Idiopathic pulmonary fibrosis
IR	Internal rotation
	Interventional radiology
IRB	Indications risks benefits
	Institutional review board
IRBBB	Incomplete right bundle branch block
IT	Intrathecal
ITB	Iliotibial band
ITP	Idiopathic thrombocytopenia
IU	International units
IUD	Intrauterine device
IUFD	Intrauterine fetal death
IUG	Intrauterine gestation
IUGR	Intrauterine growth restriction
IUI	Intrauterine insemination
IUP	Intrauterine pregnancy
IUPC	Intrauterine pregnancy pressure catheter
IV	Intravenous
IVC	Inferior vena cava
	Intravenous cholangiogram
IVDA	Intravenous drug abuse
IVDU	Intravenous drug use
IVF	Intravenous fluids
	In vitro fertilization
IVP	Intravenous pyelogram

J

JODM	Juvenile-onset diabetes mellitus
JP	Jackson Pratt
JPS	Joint position sense
J-Tube	Jejunal feeding tube
JVD	Jugular venous distention
JVP	Jugular venous pressure

K

K	Potassium
Kcal	Kilocalories
KOR	Keep open rate
KUB	Kidneys, ureters, and bladder
KVO	Keep vein open

L

L	Left
LA	Left atrium
LAC	Laceration
LAD	Left anterior descending
LAHB	Left anterior hemiblock
LAP	Left arterial pressure
LAR	Low anterior resection
LBBB	Left bundle branch block
LBO	Large bowel obstruction
LBP	Low back pain
LBW	Low birth weight
LCL	Lateral collateral ligament
LCP	Long, closed, posterior
LCR	Ligase chain reaction
LCX	Left circumflex (coronary artery)
L&D	Labor and delivery
LDH	Lactate dehydrogenase
LDL	Low-density lipoprotein
LE	Lower extremities
LEEP	Loop electrical excision procedure
LENIS	Lower extremity non-invasive study
LEP	Lumbar epidural
LFTs	Liver function tests
LFVD	Forceps-assisted vaginal delivery
LGA	Large for gestational age
LGSIL	Low-grade squamous intraepithelial lesion
LH	Luteinizing hormone
LHC	Left heart catheter
LHF	Left heart failure
LHRH	Luteinizing hormone-releasing hormone
LIH	Left inguinal hernia
LIMA	Left internal mammary artery
LLE	Left lower extremity
LLD	Left lateral decubitus

Medical Reference Guide

LLL	Left lower lid
	Left lower lobe
LLQ	Left lower quadrant
LLSB	Left lateral sternal boarder
LM	Left main coronary artery
LMA	Laryngeal mask airway
LMD	Local medical doctor
LML	Left mediolateral episiotomy
LMN	Lower motor neuron
LMP	Last menstrual period
LMWH	Low molecular-weight heparin
LN	Liquid nitrogen
	Lymph node
LND	Lymph node dissection
LNMP	Last normal menstrual period
LOA	Lysis of adhesions
LOA	Left occiput anterior
LOT	Left occiput transverse
LOC	Level of consciousness
	Loss of consciousness
LOF	Loss of fluids (water breaking)
LOP	Left occiput posterior
LP	Lumbar puncture
LPN	Licensed practical nurse
LR	Lactated Ringer's
LS	Lumbosacral
L/S	Lecithin/sphingomyelin ratio
LSB	Left sternal boarder
LT	Light touch
LTC	Long, thick, closed
LTCS	Low transverse C-section
LTV	Long-term variability
LUE	Left upper extremity
LUL	Left upper lid
	Left upper lobe
LUTS	Lower urinary tract symptoms
LUQ	Left upper quadrant
LV	Left ventricle
LV FXN	Left ventricular function
LVAD	Left ventricular assist device
LVEDP	Left ventricular end diastolic pressure
LVH	Left ventricular hypertrophy
Lytes	Electrolytes

M

MAb	Missed abortion
MAC	Conscious sedation
	Monitored anesthesia care
MAO	Monoamine oxidase
MAP	Mean arterial pressure
MAT	Multifocal atrial tachycardia
MBT	Maternal blood type
MCA	Middle cerebral artery
MCH	Mean cell hemoglobin
	Mean corpuscular hemoglobin
MCHC	Mean cell hemoglobin concentration
	Mean corpuscular hemoglobin concentration
MCL	Medial collateral ligament
	Midclavicular line
MCP	Metacarpal phalangeal (joint)
MCV	Mean corpuscular volume
MD	Manic depression
MDI	Manic depressive illness
MDRTB	Multidrug-resistant tuberculosis
M/E	Myeloid/erythroid ratio
Meds	Medicines
MEFR	Maximum expiratory flow rate
mEq	Milliequivalent
MFD	Mid-forceps delivery
MFM	Maternal-fetal medicine
MI	Myocardial infarction
MICU	Medical intensive care unit
MIDCAB	Minimally invasive direct coronary artery bypass
MIFR	Maximum inspiratory flow rate
mL	Milliliter
MLE	Midline episiotomy
MM	Multiple myeloma
M&M	Morbidity and mortality
MMEF	Maximum mid-expiratory flow
MMF	Maximum mid-expiratory flow
mmol	Millimole
MMP	Multiple medical problems
MMR	Measles, mumps, and rubella vaccine
MoM	Milk of magnesia
MR	Mental retardation
	Mitral regurgitation
MRCP	Magnetic resonance cholangiopancreatography
MRI	Magnetic resonance imaging

Medical Reference Guide

MRSA	Methacillin-resistant *Staphylococcus aureus*
MS	Mitral stenosis
	Multiple sclerosis
	Morphine sulfate
MSB	Mid-sternal boarder
MSH	Melanocyte-stimulating hormone
MSK	Musculoskeletal
MSS	Maternal serum screen
MSSA	Methicillin-sensitive *Staphylococcus aureus*
MSU	Mid-stream urine
MTP	Metatarsal phalangeal (joint)
MV	Mitral valve
MVA	Motor vehicle accident
MVC	Motor vehicle crash
MVI	Multivitamin injection
MVP	Mitral valve prolapsed
MVR	Mitral valve replacement
MVU	Montevideo units
MVV	Maximum voluntary ventilation
MWB	Maternal well-being

N

N	Nausea
NA	Narcotics anonymous
	Not available
NA+	Sodium
NABS	Normal active bowel sounds
NAD	No acute distress
	No apparent distress
NAS	No added salt
NCAT	Normocephalic atraumatic
NCS	Nerve conduction study
NCV	Nerve conduction velocity
Nd	Nondistended
NEB	Nebulizer
NED	No evidence of recurrent disease
ng	Nanogram
NG	Nasogastric
NGT	Nasogastric tube
NGU	Non-gonococcal urithritis
NH	Nursing home
NHL	Non-Hodgkin's lymphoma
NICU	Neonatal intensive care unit
NIDDM	Non-insulin dependent diabetes mellitus

NIF	Negative inspiratory force
NKA	No known allergies
NKDA	No known drug allergies
NMS	Neuroleptic malignant syndrome
NMR	Nuclear magnetic resonance
NOS	Not otherwise specified
NP	Nurse practitioner
NPJT	Nonparoxysmal junctional tachycardia
NPO	Nulla per os (nothing per mouth)
NPV	Negative predictive value
NR	Nonreactive
NRM	No regular medications
NS	Normal saline
NSAID	Nonsteroidal anti-inflammatory
NSBGP	Nonspecific bowel gas pattern
NSCLC	Non-small cell lung cancer
NSR	Normal sinus rhythm
NSVD	Normal spontaneous vaginal delivery
NST	Non-stress test
Nt	Nontender
NT	Nasotracheal
	Nuchal translucency
NTD	Neural tube defect
NUCS	Nuclear medicine
N/V	Nausea and vomiting

O

O_2	Oxygen
OA	Osteoarthritis
OB	Occult blood (followed by + or −)
	Obstetrics
OCD	Obsessive-compulsive disorder
OCG	Oral cholecystogram
OCP	Oral contraceptive pill
OCT	Oxytocin challenge test
OD	Overdose
	Right eye
OE	Otitis externa
O/E	On examination
O&E	Observation and examination
OFVD	Forceps-assisted vaginal delivery
OGCT	Oral glucose challenge test
OGTT	Oral glucose tolerance test
OLT	Orthotopic liver transplant

OM	Otitis media
ON	Optic nerve
	Overnight
OOB	Out of bed
OP	Opening pressure
O/P	Oropharynx
O&P	Ova and parasite
OPV	Oral polio vaccine
O/R	Operating room
ORIF	Open reduction with internal fixation
ORL	Oto-rhino laryngology
OS	Left eye
	Opening snap
OSA	Obstructive sleep apnea
OSCE	Objective standardized clinical examination
OT	Occupational therapy
	Occiput transverse
OTC	Over-the-counter (medications)
OU	Both eyes
O/W	Otherwise

P

P	After
	Para
	Pending
	Pulse
	Pressure
	Progesterone
PA	Physician's assistant
	Posterior-anterior
	Pulmonary artery
PAC	Premature atrial contraction
$PaCO_2$	Partial pressure of carbon dioxide
PACU	Post-anesthesia care unit
PAD	Peripheral arterial disease
PALS	Pediatric advanced life support
PAO_2	Alveolar oxygen
PaO_2	Partial pressure of oxygen
	Peripheral arterial oxygen content
PAP	Papanicolau cervical smear
	Pulmonary artery pressure
Para	Number of births in the order of term, preterm, abortions, living; see also G#P#
PAT	Paroxysmal atrial tachycardia

PBC	Primary biliary cirrhosis
pc	Post cibum (after meals)
PCA	Posterior cerebral artery
PCI	Percutaneous coronary intervention
PCKD	Polycystic kidney disease
PCL	Posterior cruciate ligament
PCOD	Polycystic ovarian disease
PCOS	Polycystic ovarian syndrome
PCP	*Pneumocystis carinii* pneumonia
	Primary care physician
PCR	Polymerase chain reaction
PCT	Post-coital testing
PCWP	Pulmonary capillary wedge pressure
PD	Parkinson's disease
	Peritoneal dialysis
	Personality disorder
PDA	Patent ductus arteriosus
PDR	Physicians' Desk Reference
PE	Physical examination
	Pulmonary embolism
P/E	Physical examination
PEA	Pulseless electrical activity
PEEP	Positive end-expiratory pressure
PEG	Percutaneous endoscopic gastrostomy
per	By
PERRLA	Pupils equal, round, reactive to light and accommodation
PET	Positron emission tomography
PF	Peak flow
	Plantar flexion
PFO	Patent foramen ovale
PFT	Pulmonary function test
pg	Picogram
PGYNHx	Past GYN history
pH	Acid-alkalinity balance
PI	Pulmonic insufficiency disease
PICC	Peripherally inserted central catheter
PICU	Pediatric intensive care unit
PID	Pelvic inflammatory disease
PIH	Pregnancy-induced hypertension
PIP	Proximal interphalangeal (joint)
Pit	Pitocin
PKU	Phenylketonuria
PLT	Platelets
PMB	Postmenopausal bleeding
PMD	Primary medical doctor

Medical Reference Guide

PMHx	Past medical history
PMI	Point of maximal impulse
PML	Premature labor
PMN	Polymorphonuclear leukocytes
PMRS	Physical medicine and rehabilitation service
PMS	Premenstrual syndrome
PN	Progress note
PNA	Pneumonia
PNBX	Prostate needle biopsy
PND	Paroxysmal nocturnal dyspnea
PNS	Peripheral nervous system
po	Per os (by mouth)
PO$_4$	Phosphate
POBH	Past OB history
POC	Products of conception
POD	Post-op day
PP	Pinprick
	Postpartum
PPBC	Postpartum birth control
PPD	Purified protein derivative
P&PD	Percussion and postural drainage
PPE	Postpartum endometritis
PPH	Primary pulmonary hypertension
	Postpartum hemorrhage
PPI	Proton pump inhibitor
PPN	Peripheral parenteral nutrition
PPROM	Prolonged premature rupture of membranes
PPTL	Postpartum tubal ligation
PPV	Positive predictive value
pr	Per rectum (by rectum)
PRBCs	Packed red blood cells
PRL	Prolactin
prn	Pro re nata (as needed)
PROM	Premature rupture of membranes
pro-time	Prothrombin time
PS	Pulmonic stenosis
PSA	Prostate-specific antigen
PSC	Primary sclerosing cholangitis
PSH	Past surgical history
PSVT	Paroxysmal supraventricular tachycardia
PT	Patient
	Physical therapy
	Prothrombin time
P&T	Pain and temperature
PTA	Peritonsillar abscess
	Prior to admission

PTCA	Percutaneous transluminal coronary angioplasty
PTFL	Posterior talofibular ligament
PTH	Parathyroid hormone
PTHC	Percutaneous transhepatic cholangiogram
P-Thal	Persantine thallium
PTL	Preterm labor
PTSD	Post-traumatic stress disorder
PTT	Partial thromboplastin time
PTX	Pneumothorax
PUBS	Percutaneous umbilical blood sampling
PUD	Peptic ulcer disease
PV	Polycythemia vera
	Portal vein
P VAX	Pneumococcal vaccination
PVC	Premature ventricular contraction
PVD	Peripheral vascular disease
	Posterior vitreous detachment
PVR	Post-void residual
PVS	Peripheral vascular system

Q

q	Quaque (every)
qAM	Every morning
QHS	Every night
qd	Quaque die (every day)
q1h	Every hour
qid	Quarter in die (4 times a day)
QNS	Quantity not sufficient
QOD	Every other day
qs	Quantity sufficient
qual	Qualitative
quant	Quantitative

R

R	Right
RA	Room air
RCS	Repeat cesarean section
R/O	Rule out
R&M	Routine microscopy
RA	Rheumatoid arthritis
	Right atrium

RAD	Reactive airways disease
	Right axis deviation
RAE	Right atrial enlargement
RAM	Rapid alternating movements
RAP	Right atrial pressure
RAPD	Relative afferent papillary defect
R/B	Referred by
	Relieved by
RBBB	Right bundle branch block
RBC	Red blood cell
RCA	Right coronary artery
RCC	Renal cell cancer
RCT	Randomized controlled trial
	Rotator cuff tear
RD	Registered dietician
	Retinal detachment
RDI	Respiratory disturbance index
RDW	Red cell distribution width
REM	Rapid eye movement
RF	Rheumatoid factor
	Risk factor
RFA	Radio frequency ablation
	Right femoral artery
Rh	Rheus
RHC	Right heart catheterization
RHD	Rheumatic heart disease
Rheum	Rheumatology
RHF	Right heart failure
R/I	Rule in
RIA	Radioimmunoassay
RIG	Rabies immunoglobulin
RIH	Right inguinal hernia
RIMA	Right internal mammary artery
RLE	Right lower extremity
RLL	Right lower lid
	Right lower lobe
RLQ	Right lower quadrant
RML	Right mediolateral episiotomy
	Right middle lobe
RNEF	Radionuclide ejection fraction
R/O	Rule out
ROA	Right occiput anterior
ROP	Right occiput posterior
ROM	Range of motion
	Rupture of membranes
ROMI	Rule out myocardial infarction

ROS	Review of systems
ROT	Right occiput transverse
RPG	Retrograde pyelogram
RPGN	Rapidly progressive glomerulonephritis
RPLND	Retroperitoneal lymph node dissection
RPR	Rapid plasma reagin
RR	Respiratory rate
RRR	Regular rate and rhythm
RSB	Right sternal boarder
RSD	Reflex sympathetic dystrophy
RSV	Respiratory syncytial virus
RT	Respiratory therapy
RTA	Renal tubular acidosis
RTC	Return to clinic
RU	Resin uptake
RUE	Right upper extremity
RUG	Retrograde urethrogram
RUL	Right upper lobe
	Right upper lid
RUQ	Right upper quadrant
RV	Rectovaginal
	Residual volume
	Right ventricle
RVAD	Right ventricular assist device
RVG	Right ventriculogram
RVH	Right ventricle hypertrophy
RVR	Rapid ventricular response
Rx	Recipe (treat with)

S

2/2	Secondary to
s	Sine (without)
SA	Sino-atrial
	Staph. aureus
SAAG	Serum ascites albumin gradient
SAb	Spontaneous abortion
SAH	Subarachnoid hemorrhage
SB	Stillborn
SBE	Self breast examination
	Subacute bacterial endocarditis
SBFT	Small bowel follow-through
SBO	Small bowel obstruction
SBP	Spontaneous bacterial peritonitis
	Systolic blood pressure

Medical Reference Guide

SBS	Short bowel syndrome
SC	Subcutaneous
SCCA	Squamous cell cancer
SCI	Spinal cord injury
SCL	Soft contact lens
SCLC	Small cell lung carcinoma
SCr	Serum creatinine
SDH	Subdural hemorrhage
S&E	Sugar and acetone
SEM	Systolic ejection murmur (with reference to cardiac examination)
SFA	Superficial femoral artery
SFH	Symphysis-fundal height
SFV	Superficial femoral vein
SG	Swan-Ganz
SGA	Small for gestational age
SGGT	Serum gamma-glutamyl transpeptidase
SGOT	Serum glutamic-oxaloacetic transaminase
SGPT	Serum glutamic-pyruvic transaminase
SI	Suicidal ideation
SIADH	Syndrome of inappropriate antidiuretic hormone secretion
SICU	Surgical intensive care unit
SIDS	Sudden infant death syndrome
Sig	Write on label
SIGECAPS	Sx of depression: sleep, interests, guilt, energy, concentration, appetite, psychomotor agitation, suicidal ideation
SIMV	Synchronous intermittent mandatory ventilation
SIRS	Systemic inflammatory response syndrome
SK	Seborrheic keratosis
	Streptokinase
SL	Sublingual
SLE	Systemic lupus erythematosus
SLR	Straight leg raise
SNF	Skilled nursing facility
SOB	Shortness of breath
S/P	Status post
	Suprapubic
Spec	Specimen
SPEP	Serum protein electropheresis
SPF	Sun protection formula
SpO$_2$	Venous saturation by pulse oximetry
SQ	Subcutaneous
SR	Sinus rhythm
SROM	Spontaneous rupture of membranes

S&S	Signs and symptoms
SSE	Sterile speculum examination
SSI	Sliding scale insulin
SSRI	Selective serotonin reuptake inhibitor
ST	Sinus tachycardia
STAT	Immediately
STD	Sexually transmitted disease
STI	Sexually transmitted infection
STS	Soft-tissue swelling
STX	Stricture
SUI	Stress urinary incontinence
SVC	Superior vena cava
SVD	Spontaneous vaginal delivery
SVE	Sterile vaginal examination
SVG	Saphenous vein graft
SVT	Supraventricular tachycardia
SW	Social work
	Stab wound
SX	Symptoms
SZR	Seizure

T

T	Temperature
T 1/2/3	Trimester 1/2/3
T3	Triiodothyroine
T4	Thyroxine
T&A	Tonsillectomy and adenoidectomy
TAA	Thoracic aortic aneurysm
TAb	Therapeutic abortion
	Threatened abortion
TAH	Total abdominal hysterectomy
TB	Tuberculosis
TBG	Total binding globulin
TBI	Traumatic brain injury
T&C	Type and crossmatch
TCA	Tricyclic antidepressant
T_c	Current temperature
	Transcutaneous
TCC	Transitional cell cancer
TD	Tardive dyskinesia
Td	Tetanus and diphtheria vaccination
TDWBAT	Touch down weight bearing as tolerated
TEE	Transesophageal echocardiogram
TFs	Tube feeds

TG	Triglyceride
T&H	Type and hold
THA	Total hip arthroplasty
THR	Total hip replacement
TIA	Transient ischemic attack
TIBC	Total iron-binding capacity
tid	Ter in die (three times a day)
TIG	Three times a day
	Time interval gating
TIPS	Transvenous intrahepatic portosystemic shunt
TKA	Total knee arthroplasty
TKO	To keep open
TKR	Total knee replacement
TLC	Total lung capacity
	Triple lumen catheter
T_m	Maximum temperature
TM	Tympanic membrane
TMJ	Temporomandibular joint
TMN	Tumor metastases nodes (universal tumor staging system)
TNF	Tumor necrosis factor
TO	Telephone order
TOA	Tubo-ovarian abscess
TOCO	Tocometer
TOL	Trial of labor
TOP	Termination of pregnancy
TOPV	Trivalent oral polio vaccine
TOX	Toxicology
TOXO	Toxoplasmosis
TP	Total protein
TPA	Tissue plasminogen activator
TPN	Total parenteral nutrition
TR	Tricuspid regurgitation
trig	Triglyceride
Triple Test	MSAFP/HCG/Estriol
TRUS	Transrectal ultrasound
T&S	Type and screen
TS	Tricuspid stenosis
TSH	Thyroid-stimulating hormone
TT	Thrombin time
TTE	Trans-thoracic echocardiogram
TTP	Tender to palpation
	Thrombotic thrombocytopenic purpura
TURBT	Transurethral resection bladder tumor
TURP	Transurethral prostatectomy
TV	Tidal volume

TVC	True vocal cord
TVH	Total vaginal hysterectomy
tw	Twice a week
TX	Transfusion
	Treatment

U

U	Units
UA	Urinalysis
UAC	Umbilical artery catheter
	Uric acid
UAO	Upper airway obstruction
UBD	Universal blood donor
UC	Ulcerative colitis
	Uterine contraction
UCC	Urgent care center
Ucx	Contractions
UCX	Urine culture
ud	As directed
UDS	Urodynamic study
UE	Upper extremity (usually preceded by R or L)
UF	Ultra filtration
UFH	Unfractionated heparin
UGI	Upper gastrointestinal
UMBO	Umbilical
UMN	Upper motor neuron
UNSA	Unstable angina
UO	Urine output
UPEP	Urine protein electropheresis
UPPP	Uvulopalatopharyngeoplasty
URI	Upper respiratory tract infection
URQ	Upper right quadrant
US	Ultrasound
U/S	Ultrasound
UTD	Up to date
UTI	Urinary tract infection
UUN	Urinary urea nitrogen
UV	Ultraviolet

V

VA	Visual acuity
vag. ext.	Vaginal extraction

VAD	Venous access device
VAIN	Vaginal intraepithelial neoplasia
VAVD	Vacuum-assisted vaginal delivery
VB	Vaginal bleeding
VBAC	Vaginal birth after cesarean
VC	Vital capacity
VCT	Venous clotting time
VCUG	Voiding cysourethrogram
VDRL	Venereal Disease Reference Laboratory
VE	Minute ventilation
VEA	Ventricular ectopic activity
VF	Ventricular fibrillation
VH	Visual hallucinations
VIN	Vulvar intraepithelial neoplasia
VLDL	Very low density lipoprotein
VMA	Vanillylmandelic acid
VO	Verbal
	Voice order
V/Q	Ventilation/perfusion
VRE	Vancomycin-resistant *enterococcus*
VSD	Ventricular septal defect
VSS	Vital signs stable
VT	Tidal volume
	Ventricular tachycardia
VTOP	Voluntary termination of pregnancy
VV	Varicose veins
VW	Vessel wall
vWD	von Willebrand's disease
vWF	von Willebrand's factor
VZV	Varicella zoster virus

WB	Whole blood
WBC	White blood cell
WBR	Whole-body radiation
WD	Well developed
WF	White female
WIA	Wounded in action
WID	Widow
	Widower
WM	White male
WN	Well nourished
WNL	Within normal limits

WO	Weeks old
	Wide open
	Written order
WOP	Without pain
WPW	Wolff-Parkinson-White
W-T-D	Wet to dry
W/U	Workup

X

XM	Crossmatch
XMM	Xeromammography
XOM	Extraocular movements
XRT	Radiation therapy
XS	Excessive

Y

YLC	Youngest living child
yo	Years old
YOB	Year of birth
yr	Year
ytd	Year to date

Z

ZDV	Zidovudine
ZE	Zollinger-Ellison
Zn	Zinc
ZnO	Zinc oxide
ZSB	Zero stools since birth

Glossary

Abscess   localized collection of pus in any part of the body surrounded by inflammation

Achalasia   rare disease of the muscles of the esophagus due to the inability of the lower esophageal sphincter to relax to allow the passage of food into the stomach, resulting in dysphagia

Acute respiratory distress syndrome   inflammation of the lung parenchyma causing a severe lung condition characterized by impaired gas exchange, the systemic release of inflammatory mediators causing inflammation, hypoxemia, and frequently resulting in multiple organ failure

Adenomyosis   medical condition characterized by the presence of ectopic endometrial tissue within the myometrium, commonly characterized with painful and/or profuse menses. Typically found in people between 35 and 50 years of age.

Amenorrhea   absence of menstrual period in a woman of reproductive age

Anemia   qualitative or quantitative deficiency of red blood cells in the bloodstream that can result in insufficient oxygen to tissues and organs

Angina   chest pain due to inadequate delivery of oxygen to the heart muscle, often described as a heavy or squeezing pain in the midsternal area of the chest

Anovulation   failure or absence of ovulation

Anterior uveitis   inflammation of the middle layer of the eye, which includes the iris and the ciliary body. It can result in permanent damage and loss of vision from the development of glaucoma, cataracts, or retinal edema.

Medical Reference Guide

Aortic dissection   a tear in the wall of the aorta causing blood to flow between the layers of the wall of the aorta forcing them apart. It is a medical emergency and can quickly result in death, even with optimal treatment.

Aplastic anemia   condition in which the bone marrow does not produce sufficient amounts of new cells in order to replenish blood cells

Appendicitis   inflammation of the vermiform appendix

Aseptic meningitis   an illness characterized by headache, fever, and inflammation of the meninges. It may appear similar to bacterial meningitis, but bacteria do not grow in the cultures of the cerebrospinal fluid.

Asthma   chronic lung disorder characterized by recurring episodes of airway obstruction from bronchospasm resulting in labored breathing, wheezing, coughing, and a sense of constriction in the chest. This can be triggered by either a URI, allergens, or a rapid change in temperature or stress.

Attention deficit disorder   disordered learning and disruptive behavior not caused by any serious underlying physical or mental disorder, characterized by symptoms of inattentiveness or symptoms of hyperactivity and impulsive behavior

Bacterial vaginosis   vaginitis marked by a grayish vaginal discharge with a foul odor associated with the presence of a bacterium, especially of the genus *Gardnerella*

Benign paroxysmal positional vertigo   brief episodes of mild to intense dizziness. Commonly associated with specific changes in the position of the head. Patient may feel out of balance when standing or walking.

Bipolar disorder   mood disorder characterized by alternating episodes of depression and mania. In some cases, it may be characterized by episodes of depression alternating with mild nonpsychotic excitement.

Brief psychotic disorder   short-term illness with psychotic symptoms that often come on suddenly but last for less than one month. The person usually recovers completely. It is a short-term break from reality.

Bronchiectasis   chronic inflammatory condition of one or more bronchi or bronchioles marked by dilatation and loss of elasticity of the walls

Bronchiolitis   inflammation of the bronchioles

Bronchitis   inflammation of the bronchial tubes; acute or chronic

Brucellosis   contagious zoonosis caused by the ingestion of unsterilized milk, meat, or secretions from infected animals; also known as undulant fever

Candidiasis   A fungal infection, yeast infection or thrush, most commonly caused by *Candida albicans*

Capillary hemangioma   common skin lesion with a smooth surface, not elevated, and well demarcated that results from an abnormal local aggregation of capillaries; also called nevus flammeus or port-wine stain

Caput succedaneum   neonatal condition caused by the pressure of the presenting part of the scalp against the dilating cervix resulting in a serosanguinous, subcutaneous, extraperiosteal fluid collection with poorly defined margins

Celiac sprue   an inherited disease of the digestive tract where the intestinal lining is inflamed in response to the ingestion of gluten, which is present in many grains including rye, oats, and barley. When affected individuals ingest foods containing gluten, the lining of the intestine becomes damaged due to the body's immune reaction. Treatment involves the lifelong avoidance of gluten.

Cellulitis   deep subcutaneous inflammation of connective tissue; often occurs where the skin has been broken from cracks, blisters, cuts, bites, burns, etc. It can result from the normal skin flora or from exogenous bacteria.

Medical Reference Guide

Cephalohematoma   collection of blood under the periosteum that usually occurs when the fetal head is forced through the birth canal. Most commonly seen as a complication of childbirth.

Cerebral vascular accident   also known as a stroke, it is a loss of brain function due to formation of a blood clot that blocks or ruptures an artery supplying blood to the brain

Cluster headache   headache characterized by severe unilateral pain in the area of the eye or temple

Cogan's syndrome   rare autoimmune disorder of interstitial keratitis that usually develops in children and young adults shortly after recovery from an unremarkable respiratory infection

Conduct disorder   psychiatric disorder characterized by a pattern of repetitive behavior where the rights of others or the current social norms are violated. It may encompass symptoms of verbal and physical aggression, cruel behavior toward people and pets, destructive behavior, lying, truancy, vandalism, and stealing. After the age of 18, it is considered antisocial personality disorder.

Crohn's disease   inflammatory disease of the digestive system affecting any part of the gastrointestinal tract from the mouth to anus. The symptoms of Crohn's disease vary significantly among afflicted individuals. Common symptoms include recurrent abdominal pain, fever, nausea, vomiting, weight loss, and diarrhea, which is occasionally bloody.

Croup   viral disease, often affecting infants, typically caused by respiratory syncytial virus (RSV), which results in upper respiratory symptoms such as a runny nose and a barking, seal-like cough, stridor, and hoarseness due to obstruction in the region of the larynx

Cushing's syndrome   condition characterized by an excess in corticosteroids and especially cortisol, usually from adrenal or pituitary hyperfunction. Signs and symptoms may include a change in appearance marked by moon facies with plethora, obesity, easy bruising, slow wound healing, and hypokalemia.

Cystic fibrosis   autosomal recessive disease prevalent in the Caucasian population involving a functional disorder of the exocrine glands marked with digestion problems due to a deficiency of pancreatic enzymes, difficulty in breathing due to mucus accumulation in the airways, and excessive loss of salt in the sweat

Cystitis   inflammation of the urinary bladder

Dementia   progressive condition marked by the development of multiple cognitive deficits characterized by a general loss of intellectual abilities involving impairment of memory, judgment, and abstract thinking as well as changes in personality

Diabetic ketoacidosis   life-threatening complication in patients with diabetes mellitus that involves three components: uncontrolled diabetes (more commonly type 1), ketosis, and acidosis, usually brought on by a stressor, of which the most common is an infection

Diverticulosis   condition of having diverticula, which are out-pocketings of the colonic mucosa and submusosa through weaknesses in the muscular layer, in the colon. They are most commonly found in the sigmoid colon, which is a common place for increased pressure and is associated with low-fiber diets. They are uncommon before the age of 40 and increase in incidence after that age.

Ebstein's anomaly   heart defect resulting in the abnormal formation of the tricuspid valve. One or two of the three leaflets of the tricuspid valve are stuck to the wall of the heart and do not move normally. With each heartbeat, some of the blood pumped by the right ventricle may go backward through the valve.

Medical Reference Guide

Emphysema   condition of the lung characterized by distension and eventual rupture of the alveoli with progressive loss of pulmonary elasticity. It can be caused by smoking, known as centriacinar emphysema, and alpha-1-antitrypsin deficiency, known as panacinar emphysema.

Endocardial fibroelastosis   rare congenital heart disorder characterized by thickening of the endocardium due to an increase in the amount of supporting connective tissue and elastic fibers

Endometritis   inflammation of the endometrium. Usually presents with lower abdominal pain, fever, and abnormal vaginal bleeding or discharge. Important risk factors include caesarean section, prolonged rupture of membranes, and long labor with multiple vaginal examinations.

Epididymitis   inflammation of the epididymis. Symptoms include testicular pain and swelling.

Epiglottitis   inflammation of the epiglottis typically of abrupt onset presenting with stridor, sore throat, breathing difficulty, drooling, and a high fever

Erb-Duchenne paralysis   paralysis of the arm resulting from injury to the superior trunk of the brachial plexus usually during childbirth. The arm is adducted and medially rotated and the forearm is pronated, resulting in a "waiter's tip" appearance.

Esophagitis   inflammation of the lining of the esophagus

Fistula   abnormal passage leading from an abscess or hollow organ to the body surface, or from one hollow organ to another, that may be surgically created to permit passage of fluids or secretions

Gestational diabetes   high blood glucose levels seen in a pregnant woman that were not previously diagnosed with diabetes

Glaucoma   increased pressure within the eyeball that can result in damage to the optic disk and gradual loss of vision

Gout   disease caused by hyperuricemia forming a precipitation of monosodium urate crystals, which are needle-shaped and negatively birefringent, deposited in the articular cartilage of joints, tendons, and surrounding tissues. The most common joint affected is the MTP joint in the big toe, known as podagra.

Graves' disease   most common cause of hyperthyroidism, it is a thyroid disorder characterized by goiter and exophthalmos caused by an antibody-mediated autoimmune reaction

Hashimoto's thyroiditis   autoimmune disease where the body's own T cells attack the cells of the thyroid; also known as chronic lymphocytic thyroiditis

Henoch-Schönlein purpura   systemic vasculitis characterized by deposition of immune complexes containing the antibody IgA in the skin and kidney, characterized by skin purpura, joint pains, abdominal pain, and glomerulonephritis

Herpes zoster oticus   common complication of shingles caused by the spread of varicella-zoster virus to the facial nerves. It is characterized by intense ear pain, rash around the ear, mouth, face, neck, and scalp, and paralysis of facial nerves. Other symptoms may include hearing loss, vertigo, and tinnitus.

Hiatal hernia   condition in which the upper portion of the stomach protrudes into the chest cavity through an opening of the diaphragm called the esophageal hiatus. It is often associated with reflux esophagitis. Common risk factors include obesity and smoking.

Hirschsprung's disease   congenital disease caused by the absence of ganglion cells in the muscular wall of the distal part of the colon resulting in loss of peristaltic function in this part and dilatation of the colon proximal to the aganglionic part

Hydrocephalus   abnormal accumulation of cerebrospinal fluid (CSF) in the ventricles of the brain which may lead to increased intracranial pressure inside the skull and progressive enlargement of the head, convulsion, and mental disability

Medical Reference Guide

Hyperthyroidism   excessive functional activity of the thyroid gland resulting in increased metabolic rate, enlargement of the thyroid gland, rapid heart rate, and high blood pressure

Hypothyroidism   deficient activity of the thyroid gland characterized by lowered metabolic rate and general loss of energy

Ileitis   inflammation of the ileum

Incarcerated hernia   hernia that is not able to be reduced, or pushed back into place inside the intestinal wall

Insomnia   inability to obtain an adequate amount or quality of sleep. It may be difficult to fall asleep, remain asleep, or both.

Irritable bowel syndrome   disorder characterized by cramping, abdominal pain, bloating, constipation, and diarrhea

Kaposi's sarcoma   neoplastic disease affecting the skin and mucous membranes, characterized by the formation of pink to reddish-brown or bluish tumorous plaques, macules, papules, or nodules, especially on the lower extremities.

Klumpke's paralysis   palsy of the lower part of the brachial plexus due to a childbirth injury to the roots of the eight cervical and first thoracic nerves resulting in paralysis of the muscles of the forearm and hand

Labyrinthitis   balance disorder marked by an inflammatory process affecting the labyrinths of the inner ear, which houses the vestibular system responsible for sensing changes in head position

Lumbar facet arthropathy   degenerative arthritis affecting the facet joints in the spine

Lymphocytic thyroiditis   see definition for Hashimoto's thyroiditis

Lymphoma   malignant tumor of lymphoid tissue

Mastitis   inflammation of the parenchyma of the mammary gland

Medullary carcinoma of the thyroid cancer of the thyroid gland that begins in the "C" cells, which release calcitonin

Meningococcemia life-threatening infection of the bloodstream commonly leading to vasculitis characterized by the presence of *meningococci* in the blood

Meningitis inflammation of the meninges, especially of the arachnoid and pia mater

Migraine one-sided headache characterized by pulsations lasting 4 to 72 hours, nausea and vomiting, and a heightened sensitivity to bright lights and noise. It is often preceded by an aura in which a patient may sense a strange light or unpleasant smell.

Multiple myeloma disease of the bone marrow characterized by the presence of numerous myelomas in many bones of the body

Multiple sclerosis autoimmune disease where the immune system attacks the central nervous system, leading to demyelination

Myocarditis inflammation of the myocardium

Necrotizing pneumonia liquefaction and cavitation of lung tissue due to a severe complication of community-acquired pneumonia

Nevus sebaceous circumscribed lesion occurring mainly on the face and scalp generally present at birth or early childhood. It consists predominantly of sebaceous glands, abortive hair follicles, and ectopic apocrine glands. It is slightly raised, yellow, orange, or light-brown with a smooth or velvety surface.

Normocytic anemia anemia marked by the reduction in the number of normal red blood cells in the circulating blood

Nosocomal infection infection resulting from treatment in a hospital or a health-care service unit that is secondary to the patient's original condition. Appears 48 hours or more after admission to the hospital or within 30 days after discharge.

Medical Reference Guide

Obstipation   intractable constipation; irregular and infrequent or difficult evacuation of the bowels; can be a symptom of intestinal obstruction or diverticulitis

Ogilvie's syndrome   clinical disorder with the signs, symptoms, and radiographic appearance of acute large bowel obstruction without the evidence of distal colonic obstruction. It is also known as acute colonic pseudo-obstruction.

Orchitis   inflammation of a testis

Osteoarthritis   arthritis characterized by degenerative and sometimes hypertrophic changes in the bone and cartilage of one or more joints marked by pain, swelling, and stiffness

Otitis externa   inflammation of the outer ear and ear canal

Otitis media   inflammation of the middle ear

Pancreatitis   inflammation of the pancreas

Patent ductus arteriosus   failure of the ductus arteriosus to close after birth

Perforated viscus   ruptured abdominal organ

Pericarditis   inflammation of the pericardium

Perilymphatic fistula   pathologic communication between the fluid-filled space of the inner ear and the air-filled space of the middle ear

Peritonitis   inflammation of the peritoneum

Pernicious anemia   form of megaloblastic anemia due to vitamin B12 deficiency caused by the impairment in the absorption of vitamin B12 from the gastrointestinal tract

Pharyngitis   inflammation of the pharynx

Pituitary adenoma   tumor of the pituitary gland that is almost always benign. Can be secretory or non-secretory.

Pleural effusion   excess fluid that accumulates in the pleural cavity and can impair breathing by limiting the expansion of the lungs during inhalation

Pleurodynia   sharp pain in the side believed to arise from inflammation of fibrous tissue; usually located in the intercostal muscles

Plummer-Vinson syndrome   disorder marked by the growth of web-like membranes of tissue in the throat, esophageal webs, leading to dysphagia. It is linked to long-term iron deficiency anemia.

Pneumatocele   cavity filled with air in the lungs that may have resulted from trauma to the lung such as a laceration, cut, or tear

Pneumonia   disease of the lungs characterized by inflammation and consolidation of lung tissue followed by resolution; may be accompanied by fever, chills, cough, and difficulty in breathing

Pneumothorax   collapse of the lung due to an abrupt change in the intrapleural pressure within the chest cavity. It may also be caused by trauma to the lung or chest, or can occur spontaneously.

Preeclampsia   hypertension arising in late pregnancy, associated with significant amounts of protein in the urine, excessive weight gain, generalized edema, and visal disturbances

Primary hyperparathyroidism   an endocrine disorder in which the body has too much parathyroid hormone, resulting in hypercalcemia, hypercalciuria, hypophosphatemia, and increased cAMP in the urine

Prolactinoma   benign tumor of the pituitary gland that produces prolactin. It is the most common type of pituitary tumor.

Prostatitis   inflammation of the prostate gland

Pseudogout   arthritic condition which resembles gout but is characterized by the deposition of calcium pyrophosphate crystals within the joint space forming basophilic rhomboid crystals

Medical Reference Guide

Psychosis   mental disorder characterized by a loss of contact with reality, often accompanied by hallucinations, delusions, incoherent speech, or disorganized and agitated behavior without the patient's apparent awareness of the incomprehensibility of his or her behavior

Pyelonephritis   inflammation of the parenchyma of a kidney and the lining of its renal pelvis due to bacterial infection. Patient may present with fever, chills, flank pain, and CVA tenderness.

Rheumatoid arthritis   an autoimmune disease causing chronic inflammation of the synovial joints, and possibly the surrounding tissue, as well as in other organs of the body. Most commonly seen in females and classically presents with morning stiffness that improves with use, the involvement of symmetric joints, and systemic symptoms.

Sarcoidosis   chronic disease of unknown origin characterized by the formation of widespread noncaseating granulomas, nodules resembling true tubercles especially in the lymph nodes, lungs, bones, and skin and elevated ACE levels

Schatzki ring   ring found in the lower part of the esophagus. It can be responsible for causing difficulty in swallowing

Sickle cell disease   blood disorder characterized by red blood cells that assume an abnormal, rigid, sickle shape resulting from an HbS mutation. The sickling of the RBCs decreases the cells' flexibility, resulting in restricted movement through the blood vessels, depriving downstream tissues of oxygen.

Slipped capital femoral epiphysis   unusual disorder of the adolescent hip in which the head of the femur slips off in a backward direction due to weakness of the growth plate. It most often develops during periods of accelerated growth, shortly after the onset of puberty.

Spherocytosis   an autohemolytic anemia caused by a molecular defect in the proteins such as spectrin or ankyrin, which make up the cytoskeleton of the red blood cells, causing the RBCs to be sphere-shaped rather than bi-concave disk-shaped

Spondylosis   degenerative arthritis, osteoarthritis, of the spinal vertebrae and related tissue; may cause pressure on nerve roots with subsequent pain or paresthesia in the arms

Spontaneous pneumothorax   sudden collapse of the lung, occurring as a result of a tear in the lung tissue; typically seen after strenuous activity, coughing, or straining

Stein-Leventhal syndrome   an accumulation of incompletely developed follicles in the ovaries that may be characterized by irregular menstrual cycles, absent menses, multiple cysts on the ovaries, and infertility; also known as polycystic ovarian syndrome

Subdural hematoma   due to traumatic brain injury resulting in blood gathering between the dura and the arachnoid because of rupture of the bridging veins. There is a delayed onset of symptoms.

Temporal arteritis   inflammatory disease of blood vessels most commonly affecting the temporal artery. It is the most common vasculitis and presents with unilateral headache, jaw claudiation, impaired vision. It is associated with an elevated ESR and is also known as giant cell arteritis.

Tension headache   headache of variable duration affecting both sides of the head; typically accompanied by contraction of neck and scalp muscles

Tetralogy of Fallot   congenital heart defect with four key features: VSD, pulmonary stenosis, overriding aorta, and right ventricular hypertrophy. It is the most common cyanotic heart disease and most common cause of blue-baby syndrome.

Thyroid adenoma   benign tumor of the thyroid which is typically solitary. A neoplasm resulting from a genetic mutation, it may be clinically silent, or functional, producing excessive thyroid hormone, resulting in symptomatic hyperthyroidism. At this point, it may be referred to as a toxic thyroid adenoma.

Thyroiditis   inflammation of the thyroid gland

Total anomalous pulmonary venous return   congenital heart disease characterized by the absence of attachment to the left atrium of any of the four veins that transfer blood from the lungs to the heart

Transposition of the great arteries   congenital heart defect in which the aorta and pulmonary artery are reversed. The aorta receives oxygen-poor blood from the right ventricle and carries it back to the body. The pulmonary artery receives oxygen-rich blood from the left ventricle and carries it back to the lungs.

Tricuspid atresia   absence of the tricuspid valve resulting in failure of blood flow from the right atrium to the right ventricle. This condition leads to an underdeveloped, small right ventricle.

Truncus arteriosus   large ventricular septal defect over which a large, single great vessel arises carrying blood to the body and to the lungs

Ulcerative colitis   chronic inflammatory disease of the colon of unknown origin characterized by diarrhea with discharge of mucus and blood, cramping abdominal pain, and inflammation and edema of the mucous membrane with patches of ulceration

Urinary incontinence   loss of bladder control

Urthritis   inflammation of the urethra

Uterine atony   loss of tone in the uterine musculature

Uterine prolapse   sagging or slipping of the uterus out of its normal position. In incomplete prolapse, the uterus drops into the vagina. In complete prolapse, the uterus may slip so far that some tissue may drop outside of the vagina.

Vaginitis   inflammation of the vaginal mucosa

Vertigo   dizziness; the sensation of spinning or swaying while the body is actually stationary with respect to the surroundings

Vestibular neuritis   unilateral peripheral disorder of the vestibular system without an associated auditory deficit or other disease of the central nervous system. It primarily affects patients in their third and fourth decades. Dizziness is caused by a viral infection of the vestibular nerve.

Wernicke-Korsakoff syndrome   brain disorder involving the loss of specific brain functions caused by a thiamine deficiency; may present with the classic triad of psychosis, ophthalmo-plegia, and ataxia; and can possibly progress to memory loss, confabulation, and confusion

Wolff-Parkinson-White syndrome   syndrome of pre-excitation of the ventricles of the heart due to an accessory pathway known as the bundle of Kent, which elicits an abnormal electrical communication from the atria to the ventricles

Zenker's diverticulum   abnormal outpouching in the upper part of the esophagus where food may become trapped, causing bad breath, irritation, difficulty in swallowing, and regurgitation

Acknowledgments

It would be impossible to thank everyone who has helped in the making of this book, but special thanks to Sheryl Gordon, Developmental Editor; Melissa Atkin, Editor; Julio Espin, Production Editor; Robin Garmise, Associate Manufacturing Buyer; Todd Bowman, Typesetter; Abhijeet and his team at Valuechain; and Nancy Gillan, Medical Proofreader. We would also like to thank all the medical students and residents who contributed their most valued mnemonics.

About the Authors

Dr. Jonathan Phillips and Dr. Nancy Herrera-Phillips completed their medical degrees at the Medical University of the Americas in Nevis. Jonathan works for Kaplan Medical as a medical consultant and a question writer and editor. Jonathan has also worked on Kaplan's revolutionary Personal Learning System (PLS) that is available for both the Step 1 and 2 Qbanks. Dr. Jonathan Phillips is a current Family Medicine resident at Latrobe Area Hospital located in Latrobe, PA, and is looking forward to pursuing a fellowship in sports medicine. Nancy is also a medical consultant for Kaplan Medical. She is currently involved in numerous projects including maintaining the Step 1 Qbank. She is also involved in updating Kaplan's USMLE simulation exams given to medical students across the country. Dr. Nancy Herrera-Phillips is looking forward to starting her medical residency in the coming year. Jonathan and Nancy live in Latrobe, PA, and have two beautiful little girls, Amaryllis and Aryana.